The ABCs of STD

A Guide to Sexually Transmitted Diseases

By

Alan S. Meltzer

With Cartoons by Robert McGee

Eden Press
Montréal - London

THE ABCs OF STD: A GUIDE TO SEXUALLY TRANSMITTED DISEASES
by Alan S. Meltzer

ISBN: 0-920792-19-7

Cover Illustration by Robert McGee
Cover Design by J.W. Stewart
Book Design by Evelyne Hertel and Barbara Steinman

Printed in Canada at John Deyell Company
Dépôt légal — deuxième trimestre 1983
Bibliothèque nationale du Québec

Eden Press
4626 St. Catherine Street West
Montreal, Quebec, Canada H3Z IS3
and
3 Henrietta Street
London WC2E 8LU England

TABLE OF CONTENTS

Chapter One
Sexy, Sinful and Surreptitious:
The Realm of Sexually Transmitted Diseases 1

Chapter Two
Germs Galore: Prevention, Spread and Control of
Sexually Transmitted Diseases. 12

Chapter Three
Gonorrhea: The Clap, The Drip or The Dose. 22

Chapter Four
Syphilis: A Right Royal Disease 32

Chapter Five
Non-Gonococcal Urethritis (NGU):
The Most Common Sexually Transmitted Disease. 44

Chapter Six
Pelvic Inflammatory Disease (PID) and Infertility 54

Chapter Seven
Herpes: A Viral Villain 63

Chapter Eight
A Trio of Nasties: Yeast Infections,
Genital Warts and Trichomoniasis 76

Chapter Nine
Lice and Creepy Crawlies: Some Common
and Some Exotic Sexually Transmitted Diseases 88

Chapter Ten
The Gay Life and Sexually Transmitted Diseases 97

Chapter Eleven
Reducing the Risks of Getting
Sexually Transmitted Diseases 104

Glossary
The ABCs of STD – A Nice Person's Glossary of
Sexually Transmitted Diseases 114

Index 118

The ABCs of STD

A Guide to Sexually Transmitted Diseases

CHAPTER I

SEXY, SINFUL AND SURREPTITIOUS: THE REALM OF SEXUALLY TRANSMITTED DISEASES

Every six seconds, somewhere in the world, someone acquires a sexually transmitted disease (STD). That means that if you are sexually active, you will want to learn all about STD — how you can get them, what the symptoms are, and what to do about them. You may think "That could never happen to me, I'm careful." That may be true, but is the person you've just had sexual contact with as informed or as careful as you are? It is only by educating ourselves and our friends that the spread of this group of diseases can be stopped. Imagine, STD are costing the U.S.A. alone over one billion dollars every year! Of course, sexual diseases are not passed on every time people make love — we have no statistics on how many sexual contacts there are in the world every six seconds, but the number is much greater than the number of sexually transmitted infections!

STD = SEXUALLY TRANSMITTED DISEASES

Sexually transmitted diseases are a very common and important group of diseases. In fact, they are probably the most common communicable diseases in humans. Where does sex come in? For the most part, these infections are spread from one person to another through sexual intercourse.

The germs which cause STD, including bacteria, viruses, fungi and other micro-organisms, are found all over the world. (These infections have been around for thousands of years, and will most likely still exist in one form or another for thousands more to come.) We can't eliminate them all, but we can try to avoid getting them. Not all of them are harmful, but some members of this group are associated with potentially dangerous complications in men, women, and children. Often these complications could have been prevented if treatment had been sought early enough. Because STD are not a particularly pleasant subject, many people pretend they don't exist. This, unfortunately, will not make them go away.

In this book we are going to talk about the most common STD and how they can be treated. Here is a list of the main members of the STD family that you will want to know about. You have probably already heard of some of them. The main villains will be discussed in the following chapters.

THE STD FAMILY TREE

Medical Name	Popular Name
Gonorrhea	The Clap
Syphilis	The Pox
Non-Gonococcal Urethritis	The Drip, N.G.U.
Herpes Genitalis	The Sore
Trichomoniasis	The Smell
Genital Warts	The Bumps

Medical Name	Popular Name
Thrush	The Fungus, Yeast
Scabies	The Itch
Lice	The Crabs
Chancroid	
Lymphogranuloma Venereum	
Granuloma Inguinale	
Some intestinal parasites	
Types of Hepatitis	
Molluscum Contagiosum	

IS VD THE SAME AS STD?

What's in a name? That which we call a rose
by any other name would smell as sweet.
— Shakespeare

VD = VENEREAL DISEASE

The word *venereal* is rather romantically derived from Venus, the goddess of Love worshipped by the ancient Romans. When it is used as an adjective describing an infection (venereal infection) it really means an infection which was transmitted at the time of "making love." Unfortunately, venereal has come to sound as unpleasant as the words "infection" or "disease."

VD is an old term, mentioned in hushed tones on rare occasions by our parents and grandparents. It has always been considered "a dirty word." Nice people just didn't mention it. Not even the family physician wanted to discuss venereal diseases. No one wanted to acknowledge the fact that VD were common throughout the local community. One did not discuss the subject in polite company or, for that matter, in any company.

To us, such attitudes seem oddly old-fashioned. Yet if you think about it, even now, in our "liberated and enlightened" times, our attitudes towards these illnesses are not very different. These long-standing beliefs and values are so powerful that the greatest obstacle to the control of such infections as syphilis and gonorrhea is the aura of mystery which still surrounds the topic of STD.

Suppose you're at a party. All of your friends are there. They all look healthy. None of them are old-fashioned, that's for sure. You can't really imagine that any one of them could have an STD. Anyway, if they did, they wouldn't hide it. You'd be able to discuss it, wouldn't you?

Not necessarily. It's a case of "love me, love my germs." Now, if you were to catch a cold from your boyfriend or girlfriend, you could freely discuss it at school, at work or at home. No uncomfortable questions would be asked. Right? What if you caught gonorrhea, a common sexually transmitted disease, from your true love? What then? Discuss it at home or elsewhere? Hardly likely! You are now in the realm of sexually transmitted disease, where superstition and taboo reign.

Let's return to the abbreviation VD. The term was originally used to describe five diseases: syphilis, gonorrhea, chancroid, lymphogranuloma venereum and granuloma inguinale. It was once thought that these five conditions were the only health hazards associated with the human sexual act. This was an incorrect supposition. From our present-day knowledge it would appear that at least twenty diseases are involved.

STD = VD + a whole lot more

So, is VD the same as STD? Yes and no. Many physicians, particularly venereologists (those specializing in this group of diseases), prefer to use the term STD since the original five venereal diseases are now outnumbered.

WHAT ARE SOCIAL DISEASES ?

When people talk about social diseases they are really talking about STD. It is a polite, acceptable way to mention the "unmentionable." Yet the use of such expressions is a way to avoid really bringing the subject out into the open. That kind of approach encourages ignorance and further neglect of the matter. Become familiar with such words as syphilis, gonorrhea or genital warts. In this way they can be more openly discussed and we can get rid of our shame and prejudice about them. People used to be too ashamed to use the word "cancer" when little was known about the disease. Now it is a common word and this goes along with our being informed about it. There is no reason for people to remain ignorant about STD.

CAN YOU CATCH STD FROM DIRTY TOILET SEATS?

You don't have to worry about door knobs, dirty cups, toilet seats or swimming pools. You will not catch STD from these. You can only get an STD by having sex with a person who is already infected. The person's race, gender, age, education, wealth, poverty, or how clean or dirty they are do *not* matter.

STD are passed on from person to person to person *ad infinitum.* It is obvious that all sexually active people are the ones at risk. You don't have to be a mathematical genius to figure out that the greater the number of partners involved, the greater the risk of getting an infection.

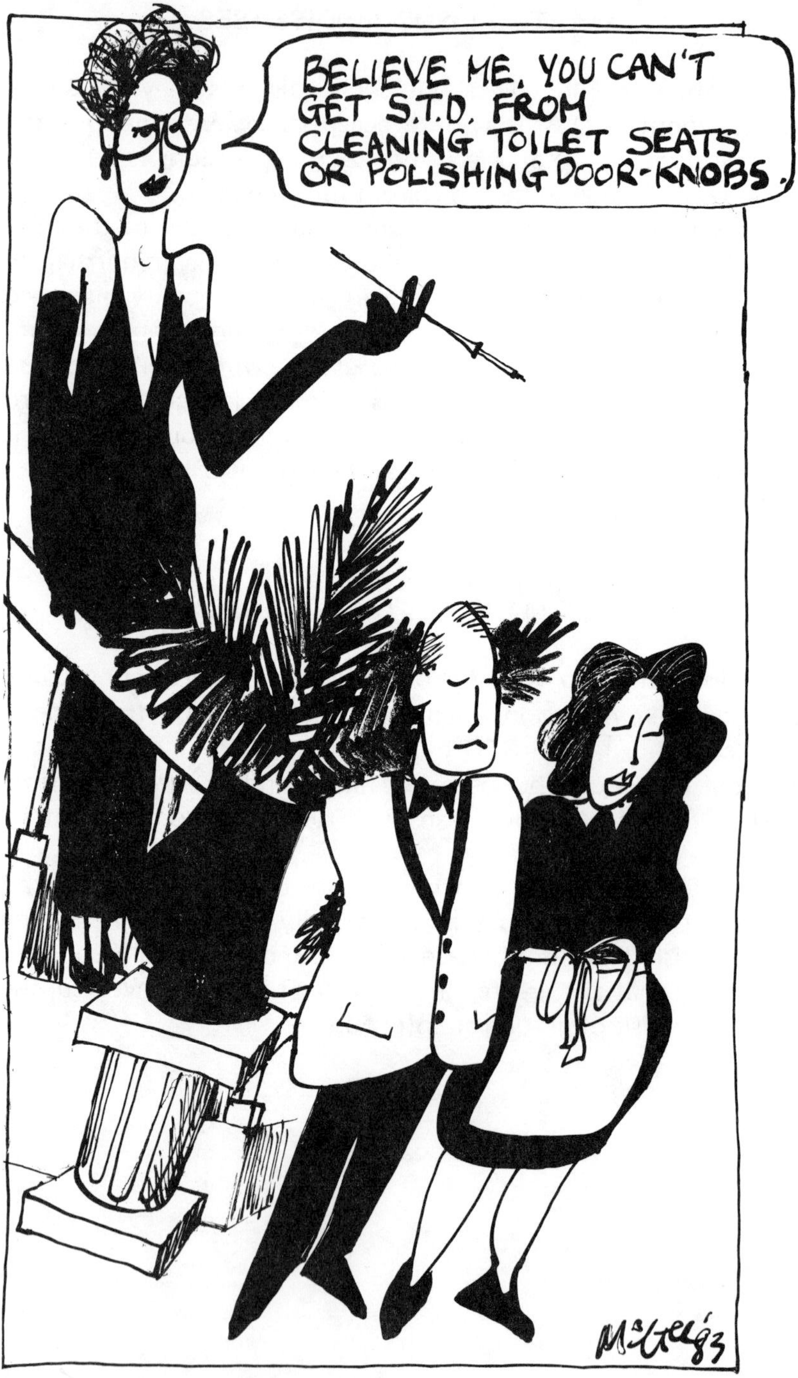
BELIEVE ME, YOU CAN'T GET S.T.D. FROM CLEANING TOILET SEATS OR POLISHING DOOR-KNOBS.

You don't have to worry about door knobs, dirty cups, toilet seats or swimming pools. You will not catch STD from these.

STD GERMS LOVE PEOPLE WHO LOVE PEOPLE WHO LOVE PEOPLE . . .

I fear they kisses gentle maiden,
thou needest not fear mine.
– Shelley (1792-1822)

What about kissing? You will be pleased to hear that, in general, this romantic custom carries relatively little risk. After all, people have been kissing each other for centuries with no obvious adverse side-effects. So, when you kiss your date good-night, it is highly unlikely that you will catch anything more than a cold, and then only if your date has one. There is evidence, however, that herpes simplex virus type I, the virus which can cause "cold sores" on the lips, may be transmitted by kissing (See Chapter 7). And it should be pointed out that oral sex (sex involving contact of the mouth, tongue or lips with the genital area) does carry an increased risk as far as STD are concerned.

Some STD, such as scabies (the itch) or lice (crabs) may be acquired by close bodily contact even if there is no direct sexual activity. Although such conditions are often associated with poor sanitary conditions and overcrowding, it must be realized that nice, clean, respectable people do get such diseases.

STD may also be spread during pregnancy. Thus, if a pregnant women has gonorrhea and goes untreated, there is a chance that the newborn child will be affected. Fortunately, with modern prenatal care, it is easy to detect and treat many STD before any harm is done.

DO NICE PEOPLE GET STD?

Yes! Anyone is susceptible to getting an STD. Years ago, particularly in the Victorian era, it was thought that poor social conditions were a breeding ground for "sexual germs" and that those who were not gainfully employed were dirty, lazy, good-for-nothings who had "low morals." This made it easy and fashionable to blame the poor, the "lower classes" for the spread of these diseases. We now know, of course, that many kings, queens, and lords and ladies of the courts also had STD. So, "nice" people get these diseases, too.

WHY DIDN'T MY PARENTS EVER TELL ME ABOUT STD?

Where ignorance is bliss, 'tis folly to be wise.
— Thomas Gray (1716-1771)

No one, not even your parents, aunts, uncles, brothers, sisters, cousins, friends or teachers ever told you about STD. Why not? They didn't tell you because nobody told them. If they did know something about the subject, chances are they were too embarassed to talk about it. Even if someone you knew had been treated for an STD, they were probably too shy to mention it.

Even health professionals may feel uncomfortable when you start asking about sexually transmitted diseases. Why all the hush-hush? Surely professionals have no such hang-ups? Sadly, they often do. Many medical and nursing schools do not touch on the subjects of STD. How can this group of infections, which affects millions of people and causes so much misery all over the world, continue to be ignored? A good question, and one that many people are asking. More and more, health professionals are trying to overcome the prejudice, and many people are pressuring universities and training centres to introduce courses on STD.

Internationally, the World Health Organization (WHO) and the International Union against Venereal Diseases and Treponematoses are actively involved in the control of STD. At the local level, most public health authorities support special clinics for the treatment of STD. The staff of such a clinic will always be willing to discuss the topic with you.

So you can see that you're not the only one who has trouble bringing up the subject of STD. This is a social problem; few people were taught about STD or to feel comfortable talking about them. As we all become better informed, it will no longer be an embarassing or a difficult experience.

ARE STD REALLY SERIOUS?

In general, sexually transmitted infections are not "killer" diseases, though in medieval times, syphilis was a dreaded disease (the "malignant" pox) responsible for the deaths of hundreds of thousands of people in Europe. Even today, in the Third World countries, this disease kills children (See Chapter 6).

If most STD are not killers, why bother with them? Aren't other diseases like cancer or heart attacks more important? A great proportion of research money and media attention is devoted to cancer research and heart surgery. Yet STD such as gonorrhea also cause much suffering to millions of people, particularly women, all over the world. Not only is this infection associated with infertility in females, but it can cause an eye infection in the newborn child which, if untreated, may lead to blindness. Likewise, the virus *herpes genitalis* affects several million people and can involve the newborn. Untreated, syphilis can have disastrous results in both the young and the old.

By now it should be apparent that STD can cause complications that are very serious and are thus worthy of our attention. We cannot hope that these diseases will get tired of afflicting humans and quietly go away. After all, STD have been hangers-on of the human race for at least five thousand years, and they continue to spread alarmingly though modern society.

STD STATISTICS

Use statistics as a drunken man uses a lampost —
for support rather than illumination.
— Andrew Lang (1844-1912)

Here are a few facts and figures to underline the importance of STD. By the time you've finished reading them, somewhere in the world, someone will have acquired an STD!

- Over one million women in the U.S.A. get pelvic inflammatory disease (PID) every year. This illness often results in poor health and is associated with infertility.
- PID costs the U.S.A. over seven hundred million dollars every year.
- STD increase your taxes.
- Ten to twenty million American men and women are thought to have herpes genitalis.
- Over two hundred million cases of gonorrhea occur in the world each year.
- Gonorrhea is becoming increasingly resistant to penicillin.
- Gonorrhea is one of the most common infections in the world.
- Sixty out of every one hundred women with gonorrhea feel well and are unaware that they have the infection.
- Untreated, gonorrhea is associated with pelvic inflammatory disease, infertility, and serious eye infections in newborns.

- Fifty million cases of syphilis occur in the world each year.
- Up to 70% of the number of cases of syphilis occur in gay males.
- Over thirty-five thousand babies in the U.S.A. are thought to be infected with chlamydia trachomatis each year.
- Over forty-five million people are tested for syphilis each year in the U.S.A.

Since not all cases of STD are reported, these statistics can only act as a quide to the true situation. Most authorities agree that the reported cases of STD only represent the tip of the iceberg; STD is probably even more common than we think.

CHAPTER 2

GERMS GALORE: PREVENTION, SPREAD AND CONTROL OF SEXUALLY TRANSMITTED DISEASES

Sexually transmitted infections are found in every country of the world. Why have these infections been able to spread throughout the human race so easily? To answer this, let's look at the factors which are involved in the transmission of STD germs from person to person.

Do these statements sound familiar?
Mary: "John *must* have given it to me!"
John: "I wouldn't give it to *anyone*. Certainly not to my best friend!"
Fred: "*I* didn't have any symptoms, so how could she have caught it from me?"

Jill: "He must have picked it up from someone else."
Jack: "It can't be *me.* I eat well and I jog two miles every day."

They could be talking about a cold or flu that they have picked up, but they could also be referring to STD. Notice how they all think that somebody else gave it to them.

It is always convenient to blame someone else. Scapegoats are useful when you don't want to feel responsible for an unpleasant situation. So goes the BSE Theory; the Blame Someone Else Theory. That's right – you never give your cold, cough or sore throat to your friends. *They* always give them to you! After all, you would never deliberately pass on something harmful to others, would you?

Obviously, this kind of reasoning is not very convincing. You have probably passed on a cold to someone else at least as many times as they have passed one on to you. It doesn't really matter who was originally "responsible." The important thing is that everyone with an infection gets better as quickly as possible. When infections pass amongst us, it is really a two-way transaction. Colds, the flu and STD spread from person to person. Now that we've firmly established that people are needed if STD is to spread in a community we must consider other factors. Do we know them all? Unfortunately, we do not.

PEOPLE, PEOPLE, AND MORE PEOPLE

Population, when unchecked, increases in a geometric ratio.
– Thomas R. Malthus (1766 - 1834)

As we all know, our planet is becoming seriously overpopulated. There can be little doubt that the sheer increase in population has made life easier for STD germs. Overcrowding has contributed to the problem. Of course, numbers alone are not responsible; what really matters is the way in which people relate to each other and how they appreciate life values.

NEW MORALS

For in what stupid age or nation
was marriage ever out of fashion?
— Samuel Butler (1612 - 1680)

We have all had some kind of religious and moral values handed down to us, been told what to do and what to avoid, who we can go out with and who "isn't a good influence." "If you can't be good, be careful" is very popular advice from friends. There are pros and cons for every kind of lifestyle, for each generation. Your grandparents and your parents may give you advice that seems "old-fashioned" and doesn't relate to the way that you and your friends want to live. Without a doubt, we cannot live in the past — we must adapt to the times and modern morals are certainly different from those of our predecessors.

Newspapers, magazines, TV and radio bombard us with information like "one in every three marriages fails," "promiscuity is on the rise" and "we live in a transient society." While these trends can make it difficult to feel happy or content, what we are concerned with here is how they affect the spread of STD. More and more people are on the move — this means that it is easier to make sexual contact with someone who is "just passing through" or just about to move away. STD can travel with them. If they leave no forwarding address it may be impossible to contact them if you discover that you have an infection. Long-term relationships are getting harder to maintain and casual friendships are popular. It may be more difficult to bring up the subject of STD with someone you don't know well. Staying faithful to one sexual partner is probably the best way to avoid picking up STD. STD can stand for Stay Tenderly Devoted.

Whatever your personal convictions are, there can be little doubt that the new sexual freedom is a mixed blessing as far as STD are concerned.

Travel is the ruin of all happiness.
— Fanny Burney (18th Century)

Not many people today would agree with the words of the diarist quoted above. After all, the thought of hopping on a plane for a vacation is an appealing one to most of us. Probably Fanny Burney did not have STD in mind when she penned her thoughts on travel, but it is true that package holidays, cruises, visits to distant and exotic lands, long weekends and business trips away from home enable people to make new friends. And this, as we now know, can contribute to transmitting STD. STD germs are real globe-trotters. People who travel around a lot can wind up bringing home unusual parasites or infections along with their other souvenirs; only to pass them along to someone else who may never have left home.

Rural-urban transfer (people moving from the country to the city) is another type of travel that is involved with the spread of STD. The city offers many more opportunities to meet people — restaurants, films, clubs, museums, for example.

SUPERGERMS

Where do germs come in? We now know that many diseases, including STD, which can be passed on from person to person, are caused by *bacteria.* These are microscopic living organisms which cause a wide range of infections including boils, sore throats, and such STD as gonorrhea or syphilis. *Antibiotics* are chemicals which have the power to destroy certain bacteria.

Supergerms is the popular label given to bacteria which have developed a fiendishly clever way of manufacturing chemicals which can destroy such antibiotics as penicillin. The correct name for supergerms is *drug-resistant bacteria.*

Are antibiotics good for you? If you have pneumonia due to bacteria which are susceptible to penicillin, it makes sense for you to take this antibiotic. If you are allergic to penicillin, taking it can actually harm you. Fortunately, there are good alternative drugs which can be substituted. If your pneumonia is caused by a *virus* — microscopic living matter which lives in human cells — it is unlikely that the antibiotic will have much effect. This leads us to an important point: antibiotics should be used carefully and only when there are good indications for them. All modern drugs have the potential for harmful side effects and should only be used when they are prescribed. Anyone who stores old penicillin or tetracycline tablets in their medicine cabinet and takes them now and then, when they feel "run down" or have a cold, is abusing the drugs. They are encouraging the spread of drug-resistant germs.

In many countries, particularly in the Third World, it is very easy to buy antibiotics and other powerful drugs over the counter. It is common for people to diagnose and treat themselves. Unfortunately, many people are not educated about drugs and diseases and they often treat the wrong condition with the wrong drug. The abuse of antibiotics is thought to be responsible for the spread of penicillin-resistant gonorrhea throughout the world. In parts of Asia, forty out of every hundred people with gonorrhea have an infection which will not respond to penicillin.

People who share their antibiotics with friends are also abusing these drugs. What usually happens is that there isn't enough medicine to go around and both the patients and their friends end up with inadequate treatment. This also encourages the spread of drug-resistant infections.

SOCIAL CONDITIONS AND STD

The link between social conditions and STD has been recognized for a long time. The great wars, for instance, have always been followed by an upsurge in the number of cases of gonorrhea. Poor socio-economic conditions are conducive to various diseases spreading through any given community. Deteriorating personal relationships, overcrowding, and a lot of other factors, such as many infections going unrecognized, compound the problem. At the present time there appears to be a world epidemic of alcoholism. There have been numerous studies and commissions to investigate the problems. There can be little doubt that alcoholism and drug-abuse exert a powerful influence on modern society which may encourage the spread of STD.

IGNORANCE AND STD

Many authorities believe that if this ignorance could be counteracted by appropriate information, then, for the first time in our history, we could talk about eradicating these infections.

How can ignorance be combatted? If all sexually active people had a basic knowledge of STD, it would be a good start; the majority of individuals who have, or think they may have, an STD usually know very little about the topic. Over the past years various "Public Awareness Campaigns" have been mounted and such measures can be useful. Many books, posters and pamphlets are available throughout the world even though most people do not read them! Mass media such as newspapers and television play a role in conveying the message to the general public. An increasing number of schools have begun to introduce the topic at junior and senior levels. There are pros and cons for all these approaches but they are a good beginning. It appears that until people realize how susceptible they are to getting an STD they do little to change their habits.

The following misconceptions are common. They show the kind of ignorance that helps STD germs to spread:

"Men don't get STD, they only pass them on."
"I'm on the pill, so I can't catch an STD."
"I don't have to worry – an STD goes away on its own."
"Teenagers can't get STD, so they don't have to worry."
"Girls don't get it, anyway."

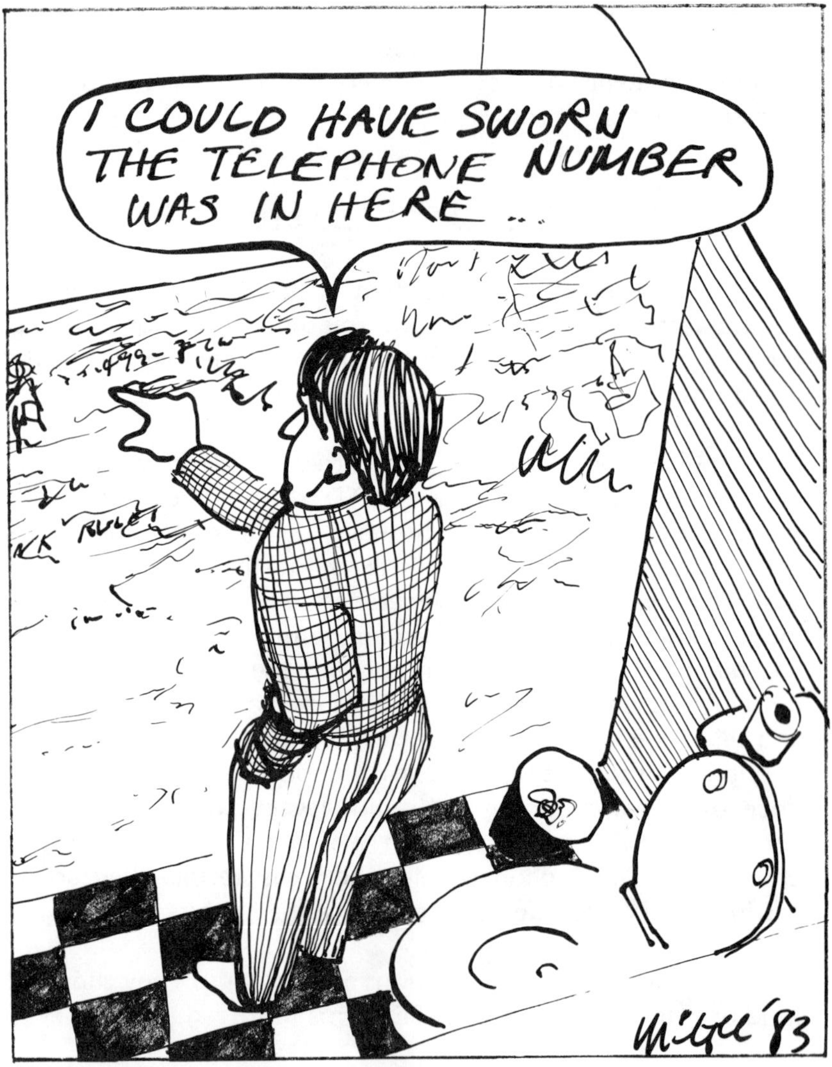

Remember contacts, telephone numbers and addresses. In the case of STD it is essential that all contacts are checked out so that they too can be treated if they have the infection.

CONTRACEPTIVES AND STD

The condom (safe, rubber, sheath or prophylactic) does offer *some degree* of protection against gonorrhea, for example. The term *prophylactic* is quite a good one because *prophylaxis* is the word used to describe preventive treatment against disease. However, the protection is not absolute and some viruses can easily cross through a condom.

Many people wrongly believe that an oral contraceptive (the pill) can protect against STD. This is wrong. In fact, the use of such contraceptives is a factor which promotes the spread of STD in that it has helped promote sexual freedom. Likewise the intrauterine device (the I.U.D.) offers no protection and can actually make some women more prone to certain types of pelvic infection. These contraceptives are effective as methods of birth control, but they do not protect the user from STD.

Another common misconception is that the cancer test for women, (the Pap test) checks for STD. This is not so. Obviously, family planning is closely linked to the realm of STD and many family planning clinics now screen their clients for STD.

PROSTITUTION AND STD

It used to be that prostitutes were conveniently blamed for the spread of STD. Nowadays, in most countries, this group of people has a relatively smaller part to play. The main concern today is with the person who has many sexual partners and who rarely, if ever, has a proper check-up.

SILENT CASES

It is important to have regular check-ups since *asymptomatic* or *silent* cases of STD are not uncommon. A person can have an STD but feel fine and be unaware that he or she has an infection. As mentioned earlier, the majority of women with

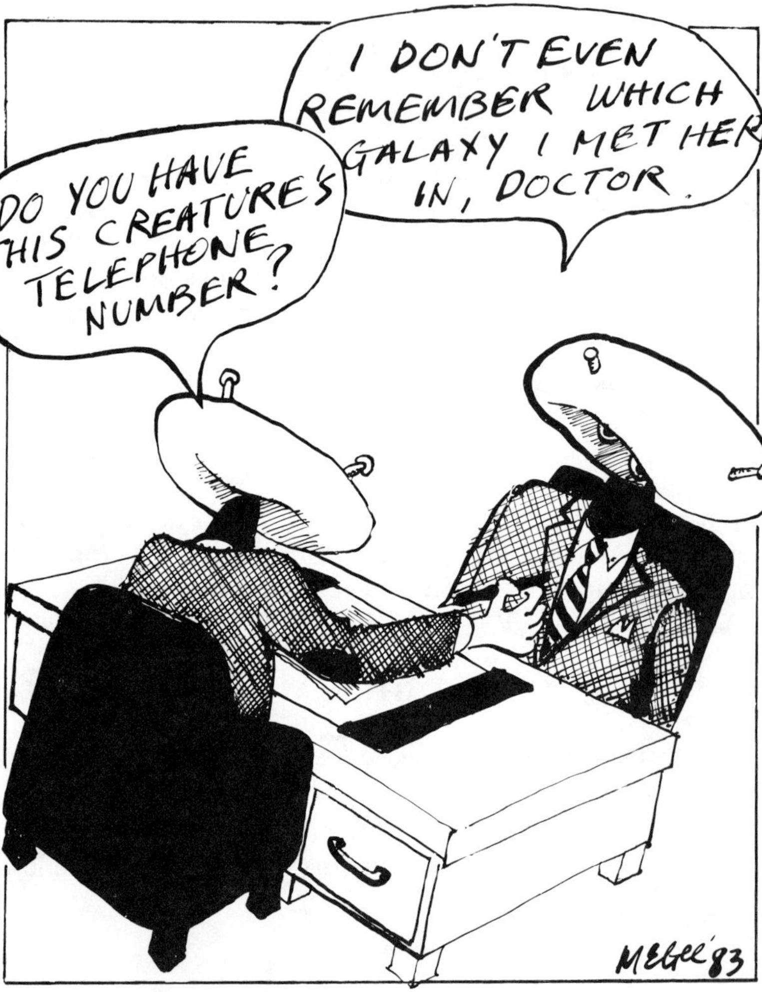
DO YOU HAVE THIS CREATURE'S TELEPHONE NUMBER?
I DON'T EVEN REMEMBER WHICH GALAXY I MET HER IN, DOCTOR.
MEGEE'83

More and more people are on the move and STD can travel with them.

gonorrhea do not feel ill and are often unaware that the infection is present. It is obvious that such a person is in a good position to pass the infection on to a partner. Clearly, silent infections are very important in the spread of STD.

LOVE 'EM AND LEAVE 'EM? CONTACT-TRACING

This brings us to the topic of contact-tracing. If a person is found to have gonorrhea, for example, then it is important that any recent partners are traced so that they, too, may be treated. Perhaps your last sexual contact was a "one-night-stand" or someone you really like stayed over and you didn't ask for their phone number. If you discover that you have an infection, how are you going to notify your sexual partner? To avoid this situation, ask your partner for his or her name, address and telephone number. This may not always seem very romantic, but getting an STD is even less romantic!

Up to now we've briefly mentioned some of the factors involved in the spread of STD. There are many more reasons, but now let's look more closely at some sexually transmitted diseases.

CHAPTER 3

GONORRHEA: THE CLAP, THE DRIP OR THE DOSE

THE CLAP: A LONG HISTORY

Gonorrhea. What a strange word, where did it come from? Galen, a distinguished physician born in the year 130 A.D., originally used *gonorrhea* to describe a flow of liquid from the penis. Galen was trained in Greece but emigrated to Rome with the "brain drain." This followed the destruction of Corinth in 46 B.C. when many Greek physicians went to work in Rome, or were taken there as slaves. Many of them played an important part in Roman medicine. Around the 14th century, gonorrhea was also called the "clap." Today it is still called by this name as well as the "drip" or the "dose."

Not only is gonorrhea one of the most common of all communicable diseases, but it is an infection which has taken a liking to humans for many centuries. In Biblical times it was common and is mentioned in the Books of Genesis, Leviticus and Numbers. Hippocrates, also known as the Father of Medicine, was a highly respected doctor and teacher in the 5th century B.C. who knew of gonorrhea and its complications. Like his contemporaries, he seemed to be unaware that the infection also affected females. In later times, gonorrhea received a lot of attention and in the 16th century, it became a fairly common condition, afflicting a great many of the European royalty and nobility.

Pestilence, fever and other severe diseases
are naught else than the devil's work.
– Martin Luther (1483-1546)

It is not surprising that Martin Luther blamed the Devil for most diseases; in those days nobody knew about bacteria, viruses and other organisms. Epidemics (diseases spreading rapidly through a community) were routinely blamed on poisoned wells, evil spirits, witches, the stars, planets, comets and a long list of other culprits. Finally, in 1879, a scientist named Albert Neisser discovered that the infection is caused by bacteria. The bacteria responsible for gonorrhea are shaped like a kidney bean and are so small they can only be observed through a microscope. They are called *Neisseria gonorrhoeae* (NG), in honour of Neisser's discovery.

To see the bacteria under a microscope, you would first have to apply some dyes called Gram stains, and then the kidney-shaped bacteria would show up inside white cells. These white cells are part of the body's immune system which fights foreign germs attempting to invade us. These cells are attracted to the site of an infection and some engulf and devour the foreign germs. This is why the Neisseria gonorrhoeae are inside the white cells. Antibiotics are the reinforcements which we sometimes "call in."

However, even though Neisser's discovery occurred in 1878, there are some people today who blame the incidence of STD on sinful behaviour and consider the symptoms of a sexually transmitted infection a fitting punishment. Unfortunately, this only encourages more of the guilt feelings and feelings and secrecy that already exist about STD.

EPIDEMIOLOGY

The word *epidemiology* is closely related to *epidemic*. Epidemiology is the study of the incidence, distribution and control of a disease in a population. After conducting extensive research on why a particular disease spreads, epidemiologists advise how an epidemic may be controlled. Here is a brief epidemiological profile of gonorrhea:

How common is it?	Very common worldwide
Who gets it?	Males and females
What causes it?	Bacteria (*Neisseria gonorrhoeae*)
How is it spread?	By sexual intercourse
Which age group is mainly affected?	The fifteen-to-twenty-year olds
What is the incubation period?	Three to seven days

INCUBATION PERIOD (COOKING TIMES)

Kissing don't last: cookery do!
— George Meredith (1828-1909)

When you first come into contact with a germ, the body "cooks" or incubates it for a length of time; this applies to a common cold, measles or gonorrhea. After the incubation period is up, things really start to happen. If you have been incubating the viruses which cause colds, you will begin to notice your runny nose, sneezes and a loss of appetite. If you've been in contact with someone who has measles, two weeks later you might find yourself covered in a rash. Incubation periods vary in length; they can last for a few days or a few months.

Gonorrhea's incubation period is three to seven days. What does this mean? If a male has sexual intercourse with someone who is infected with gonorrhea, he will probably notice in about three to seven days, a creamy discharge from the end of his penis. He may complain of pain or a burning sensation when he urinates. Of course, these incubation times are only approximate. Ninety out of every one hundred males with gonorrhea have obvious symptoms.

When you have a cold, your nose and sinuses get sore, red and inflamed, and your body's defense system produces lots of runny drips. In the case of gonorrhea, a tube called the *urethra*, along which urine passes, is involved. During sexual intercourse, the germs causing the infection invade the urethra in males and the body reacts by producing the discharge. This discharge may be white or yellow in colour. There are many other causes of discharge from the penis, but two STD are common causes: gonorrhea and non-gonococcal urethritis. You should remember that it is possible to have a discharge from the penis for normal reasons. Many teenage boys experience a normal discharge of semen (the fluid which contains sperm). This is probably due to "wet dreams."

What about females? *Sixty out of every one hundred females with gonorrhea feel fine.* Thus, the majority of women with this infection are asymptomatic, that is, they feel fine. This is an obvious reason why gonorrhea is so hard to control. An asymptomatic female with gonorrhea will seek treatment for the infection only if her partner tells her to go for a test or if she asks her physician or clinic to test for gonorrhea.

When there are symptoms in females, they usually consist of: an unusual vaginal discharge and/or a burning sensation when passing urine.

Here, even more than in the case of males, it must be stressed that other conditions may be associated with these symptoms. The presence of a vaginal discharge or burning on urination do not necessarily indicate an STD. In fact, the majority of vaginal discharges are not due to an STD. Some fungi such as thrush (also known as monilia or yeast) for example, can produce a vaginal discharge.

Urinary tract infections are often associated with discomfort on passing urine. Obviously it is important to perform the appropriate tests in such cases so that STD can be ruled out.

For both males and females it is always best to adopt the philosophy: if you think you may have an STD, do not hesitate to have the appropriate tests done. This way, you can be properly treated or even find out you have nothing to worry about.

IS GONORRHEA "LAZY"?

On the whole, Neisseria gonorrhoeae are lazy bacteria which tend to hang out in the urethra in males and the cervix in females. However, they can also be found in the rectum of both females and males. In cases of oral sex, they manage to settle down in the throat where they cause few or no symptoms. In other words, gonococcal infections of the throat are usually "silent" or asymptomatic.

How about complications? Nowadays, with prompt and effective treatment readily available, the complications of gonorrhea in men are not particularly common. Left untreated, the bacteria may spread to reach the prostate gland (a gland situated next to the bladder) and cause prostatitis (an inflammation of the prostate gland which does have many other causes). Occasionally it may produce a stricture (a narrowing) of the urethra. Very rarely, the bacteria spread throughout the body to the heart, skin, liver or joints. This may occur in both sexes.

"MALES BECOME INFECTED BUT FEMALES SUFFER"

For centuries everyone believed that gonorrhea was a disease that only affected males. Then in 1709, a book with the intriguing title of *A New System of All the Secret Infirmities and Diseases, Natural, Accidental and Venereal, in Men and Women*, referred to the fact that gonorrhea could be associated with sterility in women. This complication, an inflammation of the tubes (Fallopian tubes) along which the egg or ovum passes to reach the uterus, is also called Salpingitis or Pelvic Inflammatory Disease (PID). This condition can produce infertility, chronic ill-health, abdominal pain and backache. There are other causes for PID besides gonorrhea. PID will be dealt with in Chapter 6, but it is worth stressing the point that if females have early and effective treatment for gonorrhea, then PID and all the other complications of the infection can be prevented.

We should briefly talk about babies and gonorrhea. If a pregnant woman with gonorrhea goes untreated, there is a chance that her newborn baby may develop an eye infection called *gonococcal ophthalmia.* In an effort to prevent this complicaton, many countries now insist that special eye drops be applied to all newborn children. The German obstetrician, Carl Siegmund Franz Credé introduced the use of silver nitrate eye drops for this purpose in 1884.

HOW IS GONORRHEA DIAGNOSED?

Is gonorrhea easy to detect? Does it always show up on tests? In males the problem is a relatively easy one. The discharge which is the usual reason for a male to visit his physician or clinic for an STD check-up, will provide the answer. If gonorrhea is present, the discharge will consist of lots of the NG (Neisseria gonorrhoeae) which have been attacked by the white cells. A sample of the discharge is placed on a glass slide, then the Gram stains are applied, and the slide examined under a microscope. The small, kidney-shaped bacteria now appear red.

Indeed, the patient probably does have gonorrhea. The word "probably" qualifies the statement because other bacteria have a similar appearance. There are specialized tests to prove that the NG bacteria are the culprits.

Is it as easy to diagnose gonorrhea in females? Unfortunately, the answer is "no." In females the NG bacteria, for some unknown reason, resides in the cervix, or the neck of the womb. It is easy to obtain a *smear* (a specimen spread across a glass slide) from the cervix. However, the Gram staining is of little use for the diagnosis of gonorrhea in females because many other bacteria resembling the NG bacteria are also found in the vagina and cervix. So, another method has to be used: the *culture method.* Essentially, the culture method consists of a special broth which allows the NG bacteria to grow but prevents any other microbes from doing so. These nutrient broths are referred to as "selective media." Once the bacteria have grown (this takes about twenty-four hours) they can be identified using Gram stains. Cultures are also used to confirm the diagnosis in males.

Many women wrongly believe that the cancer smear test (PAP test) also checks for STD. It does not. If a woman wishes to be checked for gonorrhea or any other STD, she should make it clear to her doctor that she wishes to have the appropriate tests carried out. Many physicians routinely test for STD, but others only do so if the patient requests it.

IS THERE A CURE FOR GONORRHEA?

Throughout history, there have been a variety of ways to treat or cope with STD. Many of these make modern remedies, such as taking antibiotics, seem quick and easy. John Fletcher, an English playwright (1579-1625), stated that he "found the medicine worse than the malady." In his time, mercury was used to treat syphilis; this and other medicines given to treat STD, particularly for gonorrhea, were not exactly pleasant or palatable.

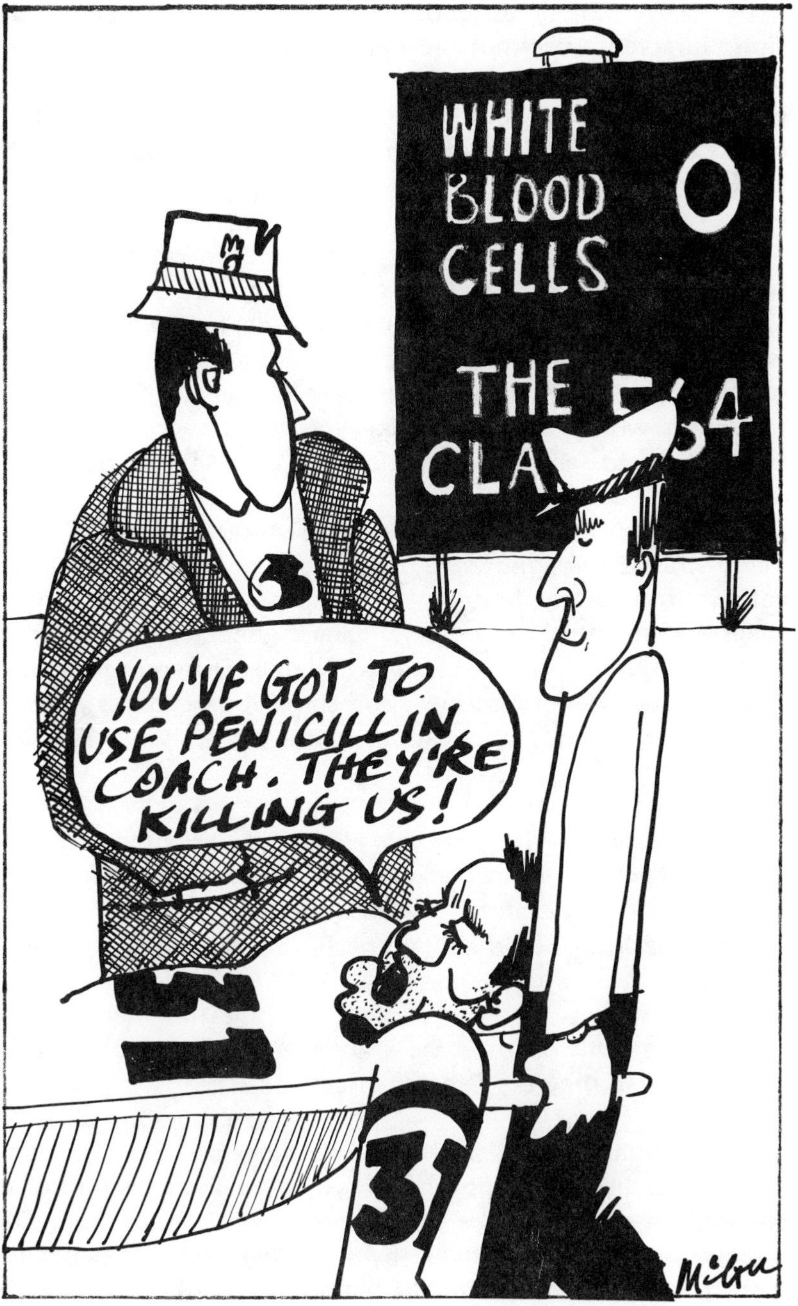

Penicillin remains the antibiotic of choice for the treatment of gonorrhea.

In Biblical times, about the time of Moses, people who were infected were put in quarantine (isolation to prevent infection spreading) for seven days. Their sheepskin garments were assumed to be contaminated too and were duly burnt. Of course along with this treatment, several doves would have to be sacrificed to insure recovery!

Hippocrates was of the opinion that "it was best to assist nature." His "doctor's orders" consisted mainly of lots of fresh air and exercise, a frugal diet, blood-letting, barley gruel, barley water, massage, hydrotherapy, and for good measure, an extract of the White Hellebore plant to make you vomit. This kind of treatment would certainly make you think twice before you succumbed to another infection, be it STD or otherwise.

In the Middle Ages, between 1000 and 1400 A.D., many strange therapies were popular. These included the application of fleas and lice, bread crumb poultices, pigeon droppings and many plant extracts. Quack remedies were rampant and there were all kinds of lotions and pills. Different irrigations and washings were prescribed, and surgical procedures were devised to deal with complications of the disease which by then were common.

In his book *The Complete Herbal*, published in 1850, the herbalist Nicholas Culpeper spoke of the virtues of the garden herb purslain. "Tis an herb of the Moon. It is good to cool any heat in the liver, blood and stomach. It stays hot and choleric fluxes of the belly and gonorrhea."

In the 20th century there are readily available cures for gonorrhea and they are safe and effective.

In the late 1930s, reports of the successful use of sulfonamide drugs began to appear. At last, after many centuries of waiting, an effective cure for gonorrhea had been found. This discovery was soon followed by the appearance of penicillin. Even today, penicillin remains the antibiotic of choice for the treatment of gonorrhea, and there are many derivatives of the original drug which are also useful. It is now possible to obtain an antibiotic in drink form for the treatment of gonorrhea. The penicillin is often given by injection but because most of us are not very keen on the idea of needles, many clinics and physicians use oral treatment.

All this sounds just fine. Are there any snags? Yes, there are. Firstly, some people are allergic to penicillin. In practice, this isn't a big problem because they can be treated with one of the alternative drugs. A more important challenge is the question of "supergerms" (see Chapter 2). In the case of gonorrhea, these supergerms are called *penicillinase-producing Neisseria gonorrhoeae* (PPNG). In parts of the world, particularly southeast Asia, the majority of cases of gonorrhea are caused by these PPNG bacteria, and so penicillin is ineffective against them. Fortunately we still have some good alternative medication, but only until the bacteria become resistant to these also.

In short, if a person has gonorrhea, the infection can be easily diagnosed and good treatment is readily available. Is that all there is to it? No. We're back to contact-tracing. This is extremely important in the case of gonorrhea where the priority is to prevent complications, such as PID in females. Another important aspect is to *confirm the cure*. We all know that penicillin is a good drug, but it is essential to make sure that the infection has truly been cured. This is done by carrying out a follow-up test between three and seven days after the treatment has been completed. The tests are the same ones used to diagnose the disease in the first place: smears and cultures in males and cultures in females.

CAN YOU GET GONORRHEA AGAIN?

The cure for gonorrhea is effective. However it does *not* protect you from getting the infection again if you come into contact with it. So yes, you can get it again.

CHAPTER 4

SYPHILIS: A RIGHT ROYAL DISEASE

WHERE DID SYPHILIS COME FROM?

To find the derivation of the word *syphilis*, we have to look back into the realm of mythology. In 1530, the poet Fracastorius described a vivid saga in his poem entitled *Syphilis, Sive Morbus Gallicus.*

On the gentle, green slopes of Mount Parnassus, near the sacred oracle of Delphi, the home of the god Apollo, numerous sheep wandered through the long grasses on a warm summer's day. Looking after the sheep was a young boy who invoked the wrath of Apollo. The god fumed and raged and as punishment finally inflicted a terrible disease on the unfortunate shepherd.

Syphilis, the name of the shepherd in the poem, became used to describe an epidemic which was spreading across Europe at that time.

The infection has always been surrounded by an aura of mystery and fear. This was justified in the past when treatment left much to be desired, but now that we know the cause of the infection and effective therapy is readily available there is no reason for people to ignore the existence of this relatively rare but important STD.

TWO MAIN THEORIES ABOUT SYPHILIS

Christopher Columbus, the Italian-born navigator, wished to find a sea-route to Asia by sailing westward, thus avoiding the treacherous journey around the southern tip of Africa and the dreary overland route. The Queen of Spain, Isabella of Castile and her husband, King Ferdinand, eventually agreed to finance the expedition. Columbus discovered America instead, as we all know. He returned to Spain in 1493, carrying a load of gold, parrots, monkeys and cotton for his monarchs. He also told of how, on the return voyage, many of his sailors had been stricken with a strange disease which caused rashes. In that same year, a massive epidemic spread rapidly across the whole of Europe. The disease was thought to be syphilis. Naturally everyone blamed everyone else. The Italians called it the French Disease, the French called it the Italian Disease, the English called it the Spanish Disease and to the Portuguese it was the English Disease.

The 15th century was also marked by numerous wars. Soldiers, adventurers and mercenaries were constantly on the march. The conquerors and conquered would often mingle once the battle was ended. Hordes of camp followers and the local people would join in the festivities. STD was everywhere! It followed along with the armies. Charles VIII's siege of Naples in 1494 was followed by another huge outbreak of syphilis which travelled on to Paris and then to England over the next two years.

Some authorities, however, are not convinced by the Columbian theory of the spread of syphilis from the New World to the Old World. Some people believe that the disease originated in Africa thousands of years ago. Indeed, it is said that syphilis was known in pre-Biblical times. Either way, the theory maintains that syphilis travelled, via the slave trade, between the African continent and Spain and Portugal, then into the rest of Europe. Originally, in the warmer climates, the infection was spread from person to person by direct skin contact. In Europe, with its colder conditions, everyone wore more clothing, so the germs causing syphilis evolved into a type of germ that was spread through the act of sexual intercourse.

A RIGHT ROYAL DISEASE

The time has come,
the Walrus said,
To speak of many things:
Of shoes and ships and sealing wax,
Of cabbages and Kings.
— Lewis Carroll

If we are to be judged by the company we keep, then syphilis is truly a regal disease. STD certainly has no respect for rank or station, and it has mixed with many of the royalty and aristocracy. At one time it was considered a normal part of any nobleman's upbringing. At the end of the 16th century, it was said that nearly one third of the population of Paris was affected. Such accounts are undoubtedly exaggerated, but they do show how easily syphilis spread into every part of Europe.

It appears that King Charles VIII and King Francis I of France succumbed to this STD. In Spain, the exaggerated and grandiose behaviour of King Philip II was explained away by the affliction. He was subject to delusions of grandeur, a late complication of the infection which involves the nervous system. The eminent Cardinal Wolsey was accused of passing the infection on to Henry VIII by "breathing" near him. Of course, many illustrious women were also affected, but, for the most part, they have been ignored by history books.

There can be little doubt that this STD changed the course of history. For example, the rantings and ravings of the dreaded Ivan the Terrible have been explained by his suffering from general paralysis of the insane (GPI), a complication of syphilis which involves the brain. This same complication accounted for numerous admissions to lunatic asylums in the past. GPI is associated with a deterioration of mental and physical faculties. It usually makes its presence felt some ten years or more after the original infection. The person is often unaware of any change, but family and friends soon begin to notice that his or her memory is failing. Work performance becomes impaired and there may be moodiness and temper tantrums. The person may also have delusions of grandeur, and boast of imaginary achievements or qualifications. Fortunately, GPI is now rarely seen.

Syphilis also took its toll on distinguished members of the artistic and literary communities. Musicians, writers and painters all fell prey to it: Alphonse Daudet, Guy de Maupassant, Heinrich Heine, Benevuto Cellini, Henri de Toulouse-Lautrec, John Keats and many other artists were stricken.

WHO GETS SYPHILIS?

Although it is not the most common STD, syphilis is probably the most important member of the STD family. In Victorian times, such complications as GPI were relatively common, and the infection was responsible for thousands of deaths each year. About three hundred years ago, if you had syphilis, you would be told that you had the "Great Pox." This was in contrast to the "Small Pox." It is ironic that we have managed to eradicate smallpox in our lifetime, yet we are still waging a losing battle against syphilis.

In the 16th century, in some countries, over half of the hospital admissions were said to be due to syphilis. The picture is different nowadays, but one interesting and unexplained fact is emerging: most of the observed cases of syphilis in the capital cities of the Western world are seen in gay males. In the developing countries of the Third World, the infection still appears to have an equal preference for both sexes.

HOW IS IT SPREAD?

By now you probably know the answer — by sexual intercourse. This is certainly true, but the infection can also be passed on in other ways. For example, it may be spread via a blood transfusion. For this reason, all blood, so generously given by millions of donors, is routinely tested for syphilis. At some stages the disease is highly infectious and close physical contact with an infected person can, on occasion, spread the condition. Also, a pregnant woman who has syphilis may pass the infection on to her unborn child. In the past this congenital syphilis was a tragic complication, associated with deformities and death. Today, thanks to efficient blood tests for syphilis, this complication can be prevented. Routine tests in pregnancy are used to detect syphilis, and by instituting early and effective treatment, congenital syphilis may be prevented.

WHAT CAUSES SYPHILIS?

Fritz Schaudinn was the son of an East Prussian innkeeper. After obtaining his doctorate at the esteemed University of Berlin, he decided that he would explore the world of germs and diseases. His most distinguished find occurred in 1905. At that time, working in close harmony with his good friend Erich Hoffman, a dermatologist, he discovered the bacteria which cause syphilis. These small, corkscrew-shaped organisms belong to a family of bacteria called *Spirochaetes* which, as the name tells you, all have a spiral shape. The culprits causing syphilis are named *Treponema pallidum.* These are small and wobble around. Also, Treponema pallidum is quite delicate, and outside the human body it can only survive for a short period of time. However, once inside our bodies it can survive for fifty years or more.

PITY THE POOR STUDENTS

Prior to Schaudinn and Hoffman's discovery of the cause of syphilis, nobody had a clue as to the true cause of this disease which had raged across Europe. As in the case of other STD, in fact, in the case of most illnesses, people found it easy to blame the weather, the planets, spirits or each other for their problems.

For many centuries it was believed that syphilis and gonorrhea were one and the same disease. In 1793, a distinguished Scottish physician, Benjamin Bell, decided to carry out a rather strange human experiment. He had dabbled in the study of sexually transmitted infections and he took pride in writing up his findings in the academic journals. This gentleman had the idea that the infection which we now know to be syphilis, could be transmitted from person to person. By taking a "jab" from the sores of a patient who already had the infection, he transmitted the disease to previously healthy medical student volunteers. Unfortunately for these poor students, the treatment for syphilis which was available at the time was not effective!

INCUBATION PERIOD FOR SYPHILIS

You will remember that the incubation period for gonorrhea is usually about three to seven days. In the case of syphilis, the incubation period is nine to ninety days. Thus, it can take up to three months for the infection to make its presence known, that is, up to three months before any tests will show positive results.

WHAT DOES SYPHILIS DO?

Remember, syphilis is still a relatively *rare* disease. In other words, most people can forget about it. Another aspect to mention is that syphilis is a great mimic; it can look like many other diseases. Confusing? Not really. If a person suspects that the infection may be present, excellent tests are available.

In its early stages, syphilis is often associated with a painless sore in the genital area. This is called a *chancre.* In addition to the usual genital sites, it may also occur on the lips, tongue or rectum. Other infections, particularly a virus called herpes genitalis, can also produce sores on the genitals and other sites. Such a condition is much more common than syphilis. Even so, most physicians and clinics recommend that all the tests for STD be carried out in such cases. Again, it should be noted that blood tests for syphilis may be negative in the early stages of the disease and so must usually be repeated after an appropriate period of time.

The primary sore, or chancre, slowly disappears over period of a week or two, but the bacteria responsible for the disease continues to spread inside the body. The next, secondary stage usually occurs about six weeks to six months later. This stage is more severe. The bacteria are reaching into every nook and cranny of the body and can do literally anything to the system. Rashes, fever, a feeling of being generally "unwell" — you name it, they can do it. Obviously, many other infections can cause similar symptoms, and in the majority of cases syphilis is *not* the cause. We have to keep a proper perspective.

In the past, syphilis achieved its nasty reputation because of the long-term complications evolving from it. These usually occurred five to twenty years after first contracting the infection. The most serious problems involved the heart and the nervous sytems, and the infection was known to cause "general paralysis of the insane," as in the case of Ivan the Terrible of Russia. However, today, with effective treatment readily available, such complications are rare.

HOW IS SYPHILIS DIAGNOSED?

Blood tests are widely used in the diagnosis of syphilis. These tests are reliable and are available to all physicians and clinics.

In 1906, August von Wassermann invented a blood test which could be used to diagnose syphilis. This became known as the Wassermann or WR test. This test has now been improved upon and replaced by the VDRL (Venereal Disease Reference Laboratory) test. Millions of people have had this test as part of a routine check-up. However, it must be stressed that this type of test is not specific. That is, other conditions, including several viral infections, can yield a positive result. This problem has been overcome, to some extent, by the use of more specific tests.

The use of blood tests to detect syphilis has been a major medical triumph as far as the screening of pregnant women is concerned. The VDRL test is routinely carried out in pregnancy, and constitutes a major public health achievement as far as prenatal care is concerned.

If a person has a sore on the genitals that could be due to syphilis, it is possible to carry out a direct test. In this test, a drop of fluid from the sore is examined under the microscope using special lighting called *dark field microscopy.* This test is positive when the corkscrew-shaped *Treponema pallidum* can be observed.

On paper it sounds like a good idea to carry out millions of blood tests, but laboratory tests cost money. Since syphilis is not a very common disease, most people who are tested will have a negative result. It has been estimated that forty-five million blood tests for syphilis are carried out annually in the United States. Of this number some one and a half million individuals are found to have a positive test. About forty-eight thousand of these people are found to have the infection. Or putting it another way, about forty-three million people have a negative test.

Ideally, people in a high-risk category should have tests on a regular basis. Many authorities now recommend that gay males, particularly those who frequently change sexual partners, should have a check-up every three months or so. Obviously, if there are any signs or symptoms of STD, an immediate check-up is indicated.

Many states in the U.S.A. require couples who intend to marry to have a blood test for syphilis. This sounds like a good idea at first, but once again, economics come into the picture. For example, in 1980 nearly five million of these tests were carried out in the U.S.A. Although 419 cases of infectious syphilis were detected, the cost of finding each case was $230,000.00 – a timely reminder that laboratory tests are expensive. Getting rid of STD would not only improve the health of millions of people, but it could also result in the saving of tax dollars.

THE TREATMENT OF SYPHILIS

Modern treatment for syphilis is excellent. In days gone by, everything and anything was used to treat syphilis: chants, charms, plant extracts, poultices, purgatives, diets, blood-letting, spa-therapy, fango therapy (mud baths), leeches, mysterious perfumes, and scores of lotions, liniments and mixtures. In the fifteenth century, mercury became a fashionable remedy. Ointments composed of metallic mercury had been used for the treatment of assorted skin conditions for many centuries. It was widely used but there was one snag – mercury is a powerful poison and the results of treatment could be fatal. Fortunately, all of the above-mentioned methods, their effects ranging from nil to disastrous, have now been abandoned.

Modern treatment of the disease began with the discoveries of Paul Ehrlich (1845-1915). Ehrlich was a brilliant scientist whose dream was to develop specific drugs, which he romantically called "magic bullets," to treat such diseases as syphilis and gonorrhea. In 1910, Ehrlich and his Japanese research assistant, S. Hata, discovered compound "606," or Salvarsan,

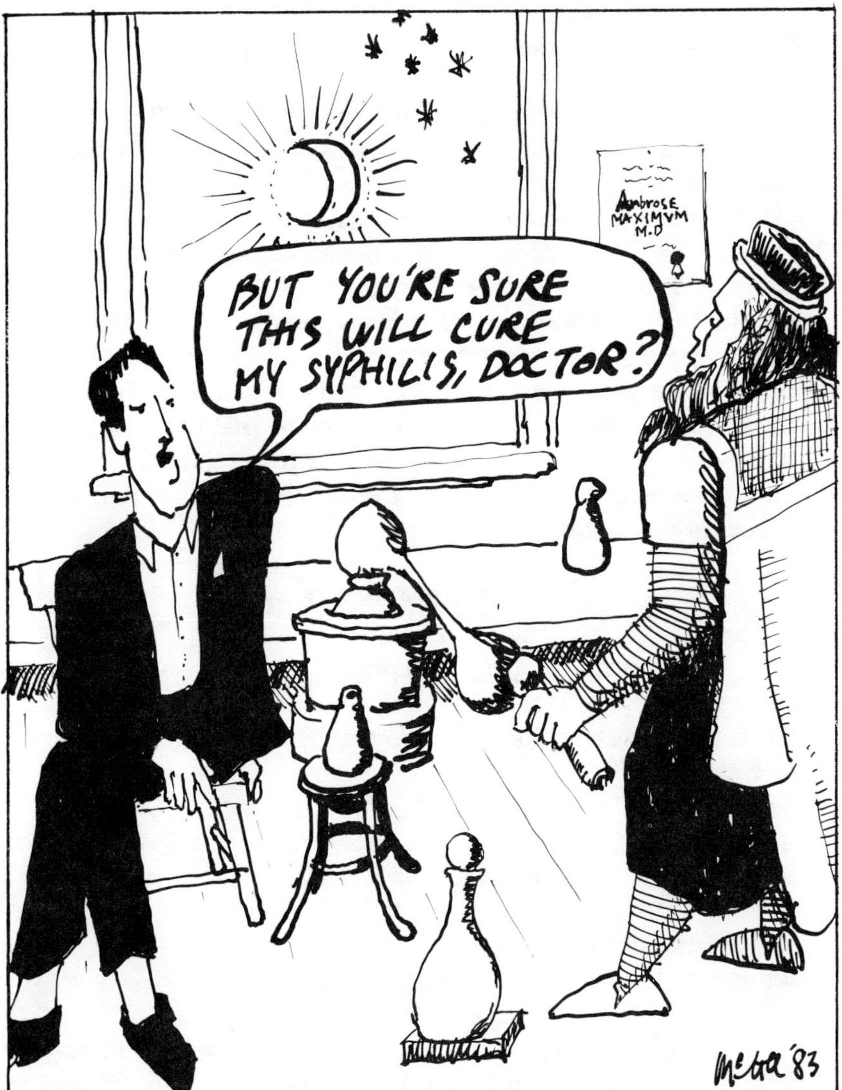
MAXIMVM
M.D
BUT YOU'RE SURE THIS WILL CURE MY SYPHILIS, DOCTOR?

In days gone by, everything and anything was used to treat syphilis. Modern treatment for syphilis is excellent.

which could be used to treat syphilis. The drug contained arsenic, another poisonous compound, and had to be used with care. Improved versions of the drug were widely used to treat the many cases of syphilis which occurred among the armies during the Great War (World War I, 1914-1918).

The next major advance occurred in 1928. Alexander Fleming observed that a mould, *Penicillium notatum,* which was blue-green in colour, was capable of killing certain bacteria. (This mould is sometimes seen growing on over-ripe fruit and cheese.) By 1941, other scientists were able to show that penicillin was indeed a highly effective drug. In 1943, J. Mahoney and A. Harris, working in New York, proved that penicillin was highly successful in the treatment of syphilis. For the first time in the history of mankind, it was possible to cure "the curse of the shepherd boy." Penicillin is still the mainstay of modern treatment for syphilis. However, it has to be given by injection. For those who are allergic to the drug, good alternative antibiotics are available.

A REMINDER

Remember contacts, telephone numbers and forwarding addresses? In the case of syphilis it is essential that all contacts are checked out so that they too can be treated if they have the infection.

HOW COMMON IS IT?

Statistics on STD are notoriously incomplete, but here is some data to help put the problem in perspective:

– According to the *Canada Diseases Weekly Report,* in 1980 in Canada, notifiable STD (gonorrhea, syphilis, chancroid, lymphogranuloma venereum and granuloma inguinale) accounted for 60% of all reported notifiable diseases. Notifiable diseases are infections which must be reported to local health authorities. The list of notifiable infections varies from country to country.

However, in many countries such infections as tuberculosis, diphtheria and the common STD are some of the conditions which are notifiable.

— In 1980, the incidence of gonorrhea in Canada was 222.8 cases per 100,000 people. The incidence of syphilis was 12.5 per 100,000. In other words, if you lived in an average town of 100,000 people, perhaps 12 of these people might have syphilis. (Of course, it could be that there were no cases at all.) On the whole, you can see from the above example that gonorrhea is nearly twenty times more common than syphilis in Canada.

— The World Health Organization has estimated that two hundred and fifty million new cases of gonorrhea occur each year and that fifty million new cases of syphilis occur each year.

CHAPTER 5

NON-GONOCOCCAL URETHRITIS (NGU): THE MOST COMMON SEXUALLY TRANSMITTED DISEASE

NGU = NON-GONOCOCCAL URETHRITIS

Well, it's not gonorrhea, so what is it? You will recall that in males, gonorrhea inflamed the urethra (the tube along which urine passes). Well, urethritis is an inflammation of this tube. Inflammation is one of the body's responses to infections. It occurs when the white blood cells (pus cells) gather at the site of an infection to gobble up the foreign invaders. These same cells are responsible for the drips which are seen in males with gonorrhea or NGU. Females who have sexual intercourse with males who have NGU often develop little in the way of symptoms. Does this mean that they are alright and will have no problems? No! Such women have a good chance of developing an inflammation of the womb (see Chapter 6, on PID) which in turn, may be associated with infertility and chronic health problems. So it is important for female contacts of males with NGU to have the appropriate check-ups and treatment.

WHAT CAUSES NGU?

The word chlamydia is derived from the Greek word, *chlamys,* used to describe the cloak worn by Greek cavalrymen. The chlamydia family of germs consists of several members. These germs are a sort of Frankenstein of the microbe kingdom for they are part bacteria and part virus. To recap — bacteria are very small, one-celled living organisms. Usually they can be observed under the microscope. Not all of them cause disease. Gonorrhea and syphilis are STD which are caused by bacteria. Luckily, they respond to treatment with appropriate antibiotics. Viruses are extremely small; they cannot be seen using ordinary light microscopes, but may be observed using powerful electron microscopes which magnify many hundred of thousands of times. Viruses are responsible for such infections as colds, measles, and on the STD side, they causes herpes genitalis and genital warts. Like viruses, the germs responsible for NGU cannot survive on their own and grow best inside living cells. The family member associated with NGU is called *Chlamydia trachomatis.*

In 1892, there was an outbreak of a strange disease among Parisians who had come into contact with parrots imported from South America. These people began to cough and splutter, to become feverish and miserable. Unhappily, one third of the patients died. The disease they had caught was *Psittacosis* (a name derived from the psittacine, or parrot, family). Although the infection is common in birds, fortunately for us the disease is relatively uncommon in humans.

So where does chalmydia fit into this scene? Firstly, the germ causing psittacosis belongs to the chlamydia family of micro-organisms. This family is responsible for several serious human diseases. Secondly, although the infection from parrots is not related to STD, early research on psittacosis enabled researchers to discover one of the main culprits of NGU.

In 1907, two scientists, Halberstaedter and Prowazeck, demonstrated that the Chlamydia family was associated with an eye disease called trachoma. (Incidently, there are about half a billion people with this eye condition in the developing countries at the present time. This infection is the world's leading cause of preventable blindness.) Following this, researchers found a way to grow Chlamydia in fertilized hens' eggs, and about twenty years ago it was demonstrated that the organism could be sexually transmitted. Since then there have been many studies linking Chlamydia trachomatis to NGU.

IS NGU A NEW DISEASE?

No, it has been around for a long time. In fact, references in the Bible describing drips and other strange conditions probably related more to NGU than to gonorrhea.

WILL NGU EVER GET YOU?

Why bother with NGU? If no one ever talks about it, it can't be very common or important. Not so: NGU is *the most common STD* in the U.S., in Canada, in Britain and in most of Europe. The situation appears to be similar in other countries, and so it appears that NGU is one of the most common of *all* communicable diseases affecting the human race.

How many people have it? This is a hard question to answer because statistics about STD are so often incomplete. Reasonably accurate "guestimates" (guess-estimates) can provide us with some clues. The World Health Organization has estimated that two hundred and fifty million cases of gonorrhea occur each year worldwide. Studies have shown that, in most countries, NGU is at least twice as common as gonorrhea.

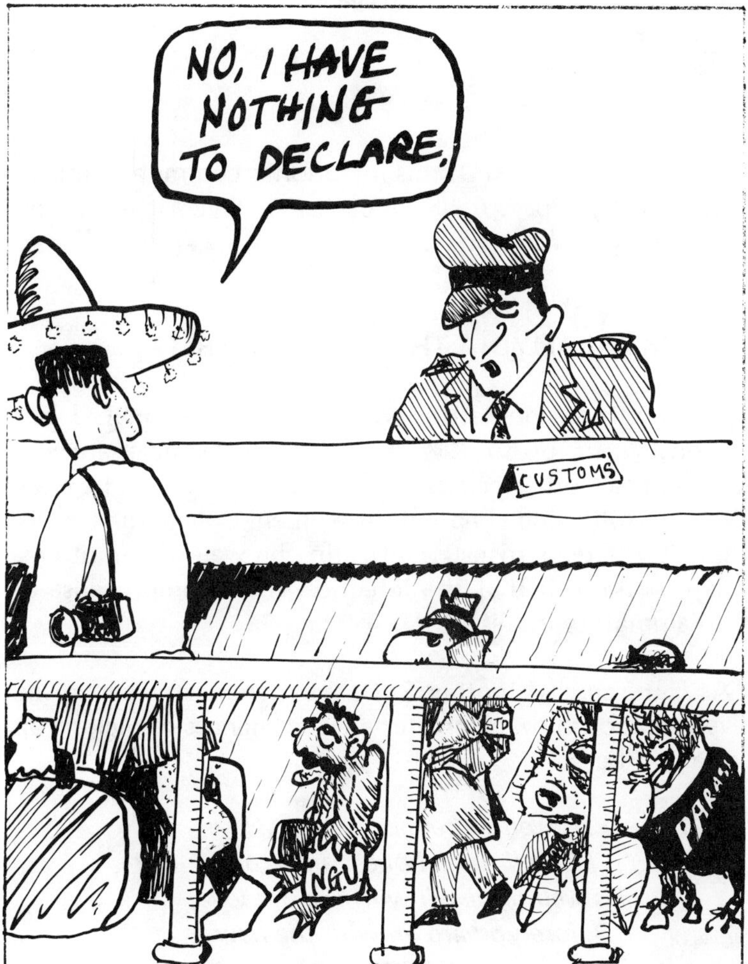
NO, I HAVE NOTHING TO DECLARE.
CUSTOMS
STD
N.G.U.
McGee '83

People who travel around a lot can wind up bringing home unusual parasites or infections along with their other souvenirs.

We can therefore assume that the number of people with NGU in the world each year is in the order of 500 million. This staggering figure ensures that NGU leads the world STD league.

WHO GETS NGU?

Like many other STD, this infection is common in the 15 to 30 year age group, but like most other STD, it is not too fussy as far as age is concerned.

IS CHLAMYDIA THE ONLY CULPRIT?

Chlamydia trachomatis is not the only cause of NGU, but it is responsible for up to 60% of cases as far as males are concerned. There are other causes, and some of these will be mentioned in the following chapters. In women, Chlamydia trachomatis infections tend to cause little in the way of symptoms, but it is now known that the infection is a common cause of pelvic inflammatory disease (PID).

As is the case with other STD, the more partners involved in a given relationship, the greater are the chances of picking up NGU or any other STD.

Tis well to be merry and wise,
Tis well to be honest and true,
Tis well to be off with the old love,
Before you are on with the new.
— 18th Century ditty

INCUBATION PERIOD

The incubation period of NGU is usually from seven to fourteen days, but may be longer or shorter.

WHAT ARE THE SYMPTOMS OF NGU?

Males will usually notice that they have the infection because of urethral discharge or drips. The symptoms tend to be similar to those produced by gonorrhea and there may be a burning sensation on passing the urine. Often, the person finds that he has to urinate more often than usual. Like gonorrhea, NGU sometimes causes prostatitis, epididymitis and urethral strictures. With modern treatment, such complications are relatively rare.

One rare complication which should be mentioned is Reiter's Disease. This illness was first described by Hans Reiter in 1917. For every hundred males with NGU, about one will develop this condition which consists of NGU, inflammation of the eyes (conjunctivitis) and arthritis. It is uncommon in women.

Like gonorrhea, Chlamydia trachomatis usually lies low in women, producing few or no symptoms. However, this does not mean that its presence can be ignored. It may produce an inflammation of the cervix (neck of the womb) but the main risk lies in PID which is associated with ill-health, infertility and complications in pregnancy. Again as with gonorrhea, a woman with Chlamydia trachomatis may pass the infection on to her newborn child in the form of an eye infection.

It has been estimated that in Western countries, about five out of every hundred babies are exposed to Chlamydia trachomatis. About two of these five babies will acquire the infection as they pass through the cervix. At the present time we do not know how many of the newborn babies will develop complications due to the infection. It was estimated in 1979 that over seventy-five thousand newborn babies in the U.S.A. had an eye infection associated with Chlamydia trachomatis, and over thirty-five thousand babies in the U.S.A. are thought to have a Chlamydia trachomatis chest infection each year. Pediatricians are now recognizing that such chest infections may be relatively common.

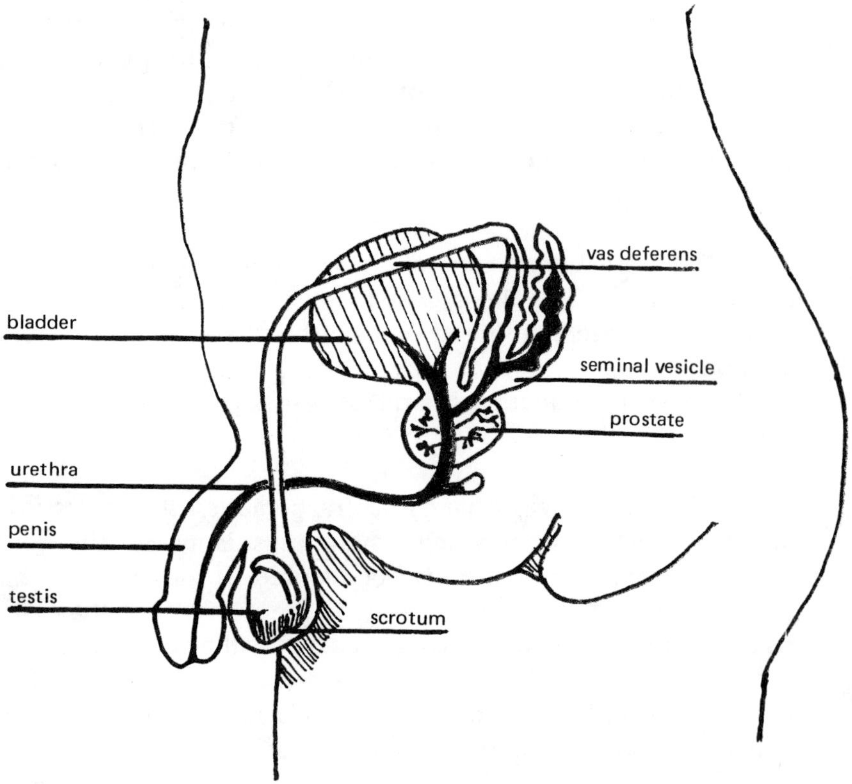

Diagram of male genital organs (simplified).

It should be noted that STD are truly sociable diseases; they often prefer to travel in twos and threes. Thus, it is not surprising to find both NGU and gonorrhea in the same person.

DETECTING NGU

Most males with NGU are "lucky" in that the symptoms are so apparent: the appearance of a discharge from the penis accompanied by a burning sensation on urinating. One priority is to ensure that gonorrhea is not present. This is done by using the smear and Gram stain tests which were mentioned in the chapter about gonorrhea. Cultures for gonorrhea are usually taken, along with a blood test for syphilis. As in all cases of STD, the physician will also take a medical history and carry out a brief examination. So, point number one: if you think you may have an STD, whether it be NGU or otherwise, have the appropriate tests carried out by a physician or the staff of the local STD clinic.

Chlamydia trachomatis can be grown in tissue cultures (suspension of living human cells). However, not only is the technique difficult and costly, but it is only available in a few centres. This culture method is the best way to identify these infections. Fortunately, the diagnosis can also be made by exclusion. For example, John, a student, developed a whitish discharge from the tip of his penis just ten days after he'd had sex with his new girlfriend. Being a clever person, he decided to go to his local STD clinic. After obtaining a few personal details ("How long have you known Jane for?" "Did you use a condom?" and so on), a slide test was made and, after a quick examination, a blood test for syphilis was also taken. On microscopic examination, lots of white pus cells were seen, but no evidence of the kidneybean-shaped gonococci which cause gonorrhea. John was told that he had NGU and that all would be well providing he took the appropriate medication as directed (in this case, a suitable antibiotic) and abstained from intercourse until his follow-up tests at the clinic were "all clear."

What about his partner? Which treatment was she given? Is it usual to treat women who have been in contact with men with NGU? Although some people do not advocate treatment for women who "felt fine," an increasing number of authorities now also recommend treating the female partners. This should be done to reduce the chance of pelvic inflammatory disease and to reduce complications for the newborn child. As has been mentioned, chlamydia causes few symptoms in women. However, when the complication of PID develops, there may be stomach pain, fever, general ill-health, backache, and pain on intercourse. A late complication is infertility.

TREATING NGU

Penicillin, which is usually highly effective in the case of gonorrhea, has relatively little effect on NGU. Now the good news. The most popular antibiotics used to treat this infection are the tetracyclines. Treatment is given orally (no needles!) and usually lasts for one to two weeks.

However, tetracycline should not be used in pregnancy or given to children as it can cause a permanent discolouration of the teeth. Good alternative antibiotics can be used.

This is a good place to mention a few "dos" and "don'ts" about STD treatment:

DO take treatment as directed.
DO get your partner involved; she/he may also need to be checked out for STD.
DON'T share your medication with your friends.
DON'T have sex with your partner until both of you have been given the "all clear," that is, told that the cure has been confirmed by follow-up tests.

There are a few other points to bear in mind. For example, as far as the treatment of NGU or gonorrhea is concerned, you should avoid alcohol whilst on treatment. Some people believe that alcohol is an irritant which may aggravate the inflammation. Another reason is that sometimes, after a few drinks, a person may become less inhibited than usual and could be more likely to have sex before a cure has been confirmed.

So, NGU is a fairly fashionable, though not desirable, type of infection to have. No doubt we shall be hearing more about it in the coming years.

Summer is icumen in
Lhude sing cuccu!
(Lots of fun and socializing,
But do not forget NGU!)
— (modified) Cuckoo Song (c. 1250)

CHAPTER 6

PELVIC INFLAMMATORY DISEASE (PID) AND INFERTILITY

PELVIC INFLAMMATORY DISEASE AND INFERTILITY

There was a young lady who was loving
with Jack, Tom, Harry and Ron
But when she wanted a family
She found she couldn't have one

PID = PELVIC INFLAMMATORY DISEASE

PID is the most serious complication of STD in females. Although it is relatively common, most people, particularly males, have not heard of it. What is PID?

Pelvic – the pelvis is a basin-shaped structure formed by the pelvic bones and the adjoining bones of the spine. "Pelvic" is the adjective form of pelvis. *Inflammatory* – inflammation is the body's response at the site of an infection or injury. *Disease* – self explanatory!

PID is not really an accurate abbreviation, for the term really relates to the pelvic organs and tissues *in women.* It includes the ovaries (egg-producing organs), the tubes (along which the eggs pass to the uterus) and the uterus (the womb).

TUBES?

The structures we are talking about are the *Fallopian tubes.* These tubes are essential to the human race. Without them, we could not have come into being on this earth. Gabrielle Falloppio (1523 - 1562) was a celebrated Italian anatomist and writer. He made significant discoveries relating to the human ear, various nerves, and he was the first person to provide an accurate description of the ovaries. This was not an easy task, for in those days one was not supposed to question the mechanics and workings of the human body, whether it was male or female. Women certainly were not expected or allowed to discuss such matters. It is only in relatively recent times that women have been admitted to medical schools or allowed to specialize in gynecology or surgery. Female professors of anatomy are still fairly uncommon in our universities and medical schools.

A CRASH COURSE IN BIOLOGY

How are babies born? The female's egg, or ovum has to be fertilized by the male's sperm, but there is more to it than that.

The ovary has the potential to produce up to half a million eggs. Not all at the same time; one single egg is released every four weeks or so. This usually occurs about fourteen days before the onset of menstruation, or about the middle of the menstrual cycle.

After sexual intercourse, the semen (male generative fluid) is deposited in the female's vagina and the sperm swim their way up the uterus to reach the Fallopian tubes. It is here that the female egg and male sperm meet. It is the fertilization of the egg by the sperm that results in pregnancy. What happens if they cannot meet? Simple – no fertilization means no baby. What could prevent this from happening? One obvious cause would be a blocked tube. This is where PID comes in.

Consider the case of gonorrhea. Bacteria causing the infection travel from the cervix to the two Fallopian tubes. The body reacts to the presence of these foreign invaders by inflammation, which results in the tubes becoming swollen and tender. If the infection is quickly cured by the use of appropriate antibiotics, then no harm is done. However, if the infection is allowed to go unheeded, then there is a chance that the tubes will become scarred. In such cases, blockage of the tubes may occur. If both tubes become blocked then the woman will be infertile. However, if only one tube is affected, then pregnancy can still occur.

The fertilized egg usually travels down to the uterine cavity where it will develop. What happens if the fertilized egg is unable to reach the uterus? If a Fallopian tube is only partially blocked it is possible for a very determined sperm to swim through any available gap and fertilize the egg. So far so good. However, since the egg is much larger than the sperm, in many cases the fertilized egg, which increases in size, is unable to get through that gap to the uterus. Thus, a pregnancy can take place in an "abnormal" site, the Fallopian tube. (This is called an ectopic pregnancy.) In such cases the lives of both mother and baby are at risk. Emergency surgery is often required and there is also a risk of severe hemorrhaging. In many countries, the incidence of these ectopic pregnancies appears to be increasing, and in many cases PID is the real cause. This is a shame, because most cases of PID are preventable.

PID IS THE MOST SERIOUS COMPLICATION OF STD IN FEMALES

WHAT CAUSES PID?

There are many causes. As you may have guessed by now, many of them are members of the STD family. The two main villains are Neisseria gonorrhoeae (the bacteria causing gonorrhea) and Chlamydia trachomatis (a common cause of non-gonococcal urethritis – NGU). However, it should be stressed that other conditions may be associated with PID.

Remember, most males with gonorrhea and/or NGU *have* symptoms and most females with gonorrhea and/or NGU have *no* symptoms. In other words, the majority of males with these types of STD know that "something is wrong" and can seek medical assistance, BUT, and it is a big but – most of their female partners feel just fine and so will not seek any medical assistance unless their male partners let them know what's happening.

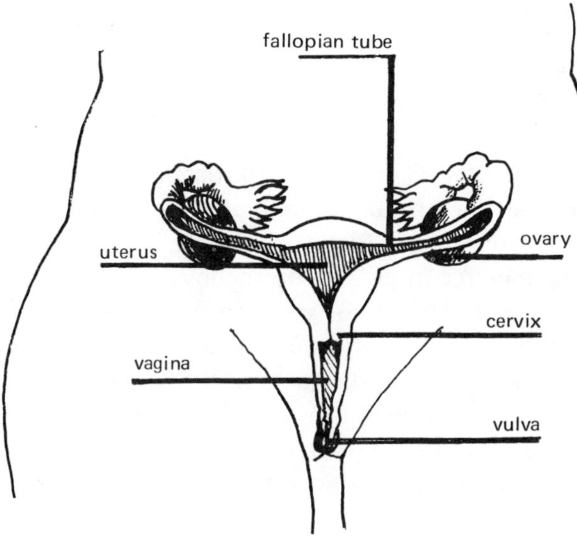

Diagram of female genital organs (simplified).

What happens if these women do not go for a check-up? Well, for starters, it is known that ten to fifteen percent of these women will develop PID (and this could have been prevented if they had received treatment at the *same time as their male partners*). Also, they are liable to develop the other complications of gonorrhea and Chlamydia trachomatis infections. In addition, their partners will become reinfected, and if they are pregnant, there is a good chance that the newborn baby will become infected.

WHAT ARE THE SYMPTOMS OF PID?

— pain in the abdomen
— fever
— ill-health
— fatigue
— backache
— pain on intercourse
— vaginal discharge
— heavy periods
— nausea
— vomiting
— infertility
— nothing may be noticed, i.e., the female may "feel fine"

Mild cases of PID may go unnoticed. Sometimes the person may be aware of a mild stomach ache. Any long-standing infection can cause fever, fatigue, and a feeling of being unwell. Severe cases may result in an emergency, requiring immediate admission to hospital. Obviously, there are other causes of these symptoms, and in particular, abdominal pain, fever, vaginal discharge, vomiting and other features of PID may be due to other conditions. So, in all cases it is essential to rule out other causes, especially since PID may mimic acute appendicitis, twisted ovary, bowel problems, kidney infections, and a host of other conditions.

The IUD (intrauterine device) contraceptive "sits" in the cavity of the uterus and predisposes some women to PID. Some studies have shown that IUD users are three times more likely to develop PID than non-IUD users. Interestingly enough, there is some suggestion that the oral contraceptive (the pill) offers a slight protection against PID (but *not*, of course, against STD).

INFERTILITY

There was an old woman who lived in a shoe,
She had so many children she didn't know what to do.

The woman in the nursery rhyme certainly did not suffer from infertility. Infertility really means "failing to produce offspring." Many couples do not wish to have children, and this is a different state of affairs. Other couples wish to have a family but are unable to do so. Sometimes the reason for this childlessness lies with the male partner and sometimes it lies with the female. Here we are only concerned with infertility due to PID. This is one of the most serious complications of PID. Indeed, some people refer to PID as the Popular Infertility Device.

In West Africa there is a group of villages in the middle of dense tropical vegetation. The air is hot and humid. The visitor soon notices that the houses, or more accurately, the mud huts, are small and that overcrowding is the rule. The people have no water and can only obtain this precious commodity by walking through the bush to the unreliable shallow well some six kilometres away. Soon the visitor becomes aware of how quiet it is. No children can be seen wandering through the villages. The young women all appear to be very serious and only the rare one can be seen carrying a young child. The village elder solemnly tells how the village population appears to be dwindling. A strange situation indeed.

These villages do exist in many areas of tropical Africa. Why are there so few children? Nearly half of these village

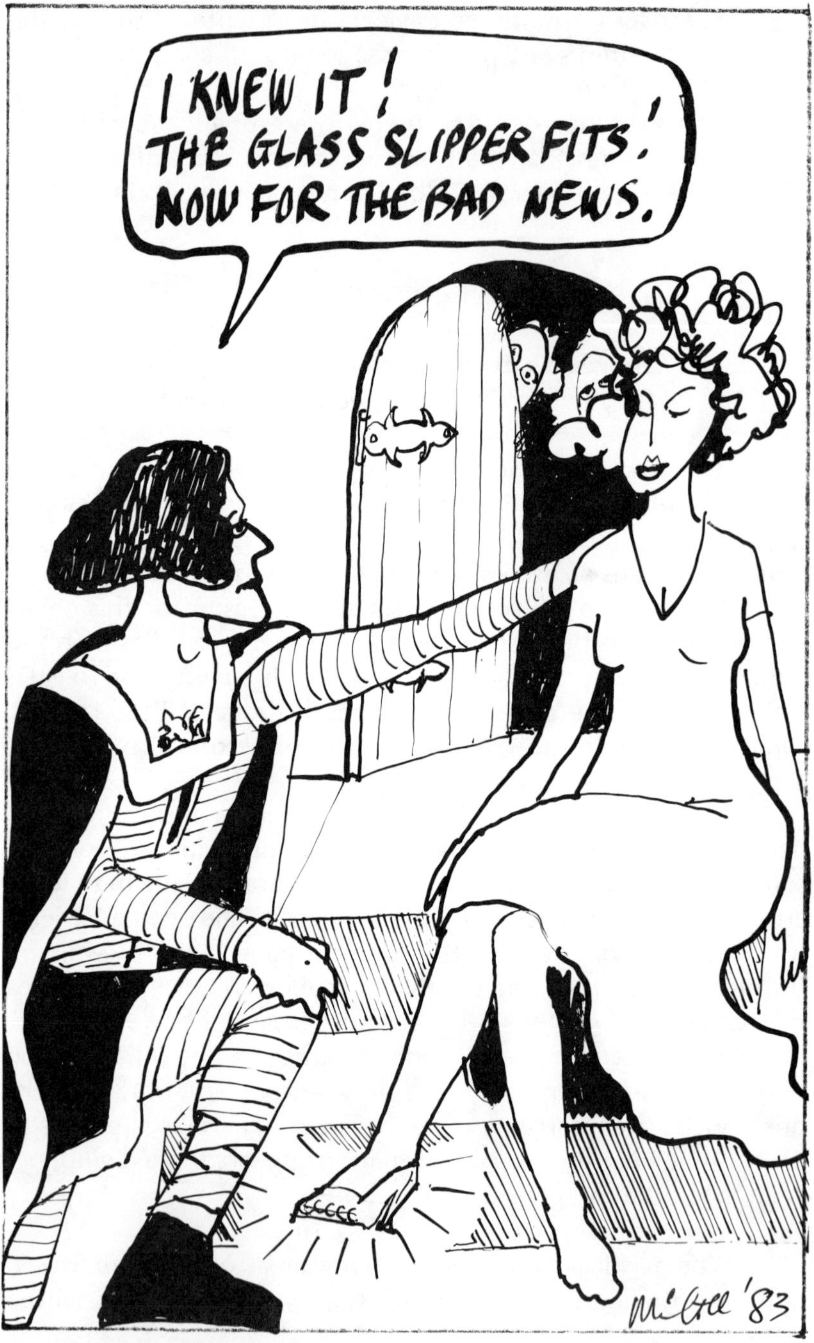
I KNEW IT!
THE GLASS SLIPPER FITS!
NOW FOR THE BAD NEWS.

The incidence of PID would be reduced if males would let their female partners know when they have an STD.

women are infertile because of PID which was caused by STD. Most of it could have been prevented!

In the western world infertility due to STD, and PID in particular, appears to be on the increase as well. It has been estimated that by the year 2000, more and more young women between the ages of 18 (and younger) and 25 will be infertile, and this will be a significant problem.

Should we worry? After all, they are developing the technology of the "test-tube baby." Well, this is a clever technical trick, and an impressive one, but it is not without risk and there are many legal and ethical implications. To merely implant the fertilized egg into the mother does not necessarily avert any contact the baby might have with STD as the child can become infected during the birth itself. A much better approach to the problem of infertility is to prevent PID in women by treating and controlling STD.

A GRAM OF PREVENTION
IS WORTH A KILOGRAM OF CURE

Because most males with STD have symptoms and thus usually have early antibiotic treatment, infertility is now relatively rare in men with STD.

DISTURBING FACTS

If a woman has PID, how high is the actual risk of her becoming infertile? Because of the many variables involved, it is not possible to come up with exact figures for each specific situation. For example, much depends upon how soon therapy is instituted. However, studies have shown the following tendencies:

After the *first* episode of PID there is a 12% chance of infertility.

After the *second* episode of PID there is a 36% chance of infertility.
After the *third* episode of PID there is a 72% chance of infertility.

This is not the whole story, for women who have had PID have a greater risk at having an ectopic pregnancy when they do get pregnant.

PID IS PROBABLY THE MOST COMMON CAUSE OF INFERTILITY TODAY

Not only does PID cause much suffering and misery, but it also has important economic implications:

1. In 1979, PID and its complications cost the U.S.A. over one billion dollars.
2. Over one million cases of PID occur each year in the U.S.A. (This is virtually an epidemic.)
3. The majority of the cases of PID in the U.S.A. are associated with STD.
4. Over half of the women hospitalized with PID in the U.S.A. were under the age of 25, and most were unmarried and childless.
5. Over two hundred and fifty thousand women are admitted to hospital with PID each year in the U.S.A.
6. More than forty thousand ectopic pregnancies occur in the U.S.A. each year, and most of these pregnancies are associated with PID.
7. More than fifty thousand American women undergo surgery each year because of PID.

So PID causes misery, suffering, ill-health, infertility, hospitalization, complications requiring surgery, and costs millions of dollars every year. Sadly enough, *most cases could have been prevented.*

CHAPTER 7

HERPES: A VIRAL VILLAIN

A strange viral villain, popularly known as herpes, has chosen to live securely within our bodies, emerging from time to time to pursue its nefarious activities. That is, a person who has been infected with the herpes virus may have no symptoms for months at a time, then will experience an outbreak.

As we have already mentioned, viruses are minute bits of living matter which cannot survive on their own and so they prey on living cells. Measles, colds, influenza and warts are a few of the miserable conditions that viruses inflict upon us.

Herpes belongs to a family of viruses whose members cause chicken-pox, shingles and infectious mononucleosis as well as other infections. Although the herpes virus was first identified in 1960, we still don't know too much about it. We do know that it is an extremely active entity.

IS HERPES AN STD?

Herpes is not always transmitted sexually. We are all familiar with "cold sores" on the lips. These are properly named *herpes labialis* (Latin, *labia* – lips) and are caused by herpes simplex virus type I. The infection appears to spread mainly though the act of kissing and is found in all age groups.

Herpes simplex virus type II is a very close relative, almost an identical twin, of the virus which invades our lips. It is the viral villain which is associated with the sexually transmitted herpes genitalis. Herpes genitalis produces "cold sores" in the genital area of both sexes.

Can these two viruses raid each others' territory? In the past it was believed that herpes simplex virus type I only produced infections above the level of the waist, particularly on the lips, while type II herpes was thought only to involve the genital area. We now know that this is not the case. The two viruses *can* readily interchange roles. Some clinical studies in university students have shown that the type I virus may be responsible for nearly one third of genital infections. Kissing and oral sex are factors in such cases.

Some people may ask "Did I get my cold sore on the lips through sex?" This is a common question. In the majority of cases the answer is no. However, let us just spend a minute on this aspect. It has been estimated that over twenty million people suffer from cold sores on the lips each year. So, the herpes virus certainly gets around! The virus is passed on from person to person by the act of kissing. Even an innocent kiss from an aunt to her adoring niece or nephew may help to spread the virus around. Following the first episode, the virus lies low, waiting to flare up again. Recurrences tend to take place after exposure to the sun, or when a person is generally rundown because of ill-health or stress. Returning to our question at the beginning of this paragraph, the answer is that although some cases of cold sores on the lips may be related to sexual activity, in the majority of cases the "innocent" kiss is the culprit. So, people with an active cold sore on the lips should postpone any kissing until the cold sore has departed. Now let us return to the herpes virus which is spread through sexual intercourse.

WHAT DOES "HERPES" MEAN?

The French physician Jean Astruc named the infection in the eighteenth century. He derived the name from the Greek word for "creeping" – *herpes.* The name is an apt one, for the virus creeps along nerves to reach the skin surface, and the lesions it produces often leave a snake-like trail along the skin.

The herpes virus hides away in a safe retreat in a bundle of nerves deep inside our bodies. Periodically, the virus ventures out by passing along to nerve fibre to reach the skin in the genital area (around the penis in males, and around the skin surrounding the vagina and around the vagina itself in females). There the virus multiplies and causes a rash of painful blisters, causing the infected person to feel generally unwell for a day or two. The lesions usually last for one to three weeks. Then presto! They disappear. Has the virus really gone for good? In two-thirds of the cases the herpes virus has merely crept back along a nerve to reach a safe hideaway where it can go undetected. Later, after a period of months or even years, it will repeat the sequence, once again advancing along the nerves to reach the skin in the genital area.

Why does the virus advance and retreat? While it is producing blisters in the skin, it is ensuring that it will have the chance to survive. Each blister contains millions of viruses. The virus has to make contact with another human being, otherwise, when the host (the person carrying the virus) dies, so does the virus. The herpes virus has evolved into a sexually transmitted disease as a means of spreading. By retreating back along the nerves the virus gives itself another chance to infect someone else at a later date.

Fortunately for the majority of people who have recurrences, each successive attack tends to become milder and occurs at less frequent intervals. However, herpes probably has the best survival mechanism of any infectious agent. In some cases the infection lasts for twenty to thirty years.

INCUBATION PERIOD FOR HERPES

Have sex in haste, repent at leisure.
— modified 18th Century saying

If a person acquires herpes for the first time, how long does it take until the infection makes its presence felt?

Jerry and Jennifer had spent a wonderful summer together. They had the same interests and got on well with each other. Life was great. They planned to spend a few days away at the coast. Two days before their departure, Jerry began to be aware of a burning sensation on his penis. "Should shower more often," he muttered to himself. The next morning he awoke to find a few small, reddish blisters on his penis. He was alarmed and decided to talk with Jennifer about it. They wisely agreed to delay their planned vacation until they found out what the symptoms meant. Jennifer remembered a film she had seen in high school. She hadn't paid too much attention at the time but she did remember that sores or anything unusual in the genital area could mean an STD. Jerry decided to visit his family doctor that day. After an examination and after the appropriate tests had been made, Jerry was informed that herpes was the likely culprit. Jennifer was also advised to have a check-up. She agreed immediately. How did Jerry pick up the virus? We should mention that his previous girlfriend had complained of blisters around the vagina from time to time.

Now, back to the question of the incubation period for herpes. What would have happened if Jerry had ignored the situation or been too embarassed to tell Jennifer and had sex with her on their vacation. There would have been a good chance that Jennifer would have developed the tell-tale blisters about four to six days later. To put it another way, the incubation period of herpes genitalis ranges from four to six days.

IS HERPES THAT HARMFUL?

The old prejudices and taboos associated with STD have a field day as far as herpes is concerned. Unfortunately, these have caused much unnecessary anxiety to many people. A more optimistic approach is certainly warranted; particularly since modern research into the infection is now producing improved treatment.

What actually happens when a person first gets herpes? In many cases the onset is signified by fever, headaches, fatigue, and generally "feeling rotten." A burning or itchy sensation in the genital area usually follows. Less often, the anal area is involved. A day or two later, a group of small blisters, up to two millimetres in diameter, make their unwelcome appearance. These blisters contain millions of infectious viruses. Later, they will burst to spill their contents. At this stage they hope that their human host, male or female, will cooperate by having sex with another person so that the infection can be spread. Luckily, we now know that this is the one time *not* to have intercourse if the spread of the infection is to be halted. At this stage the skin lesions become painful. In females the discomfort may be severe enough to interfere with the passage of urine. By this time most people with herpes will also notice a few small, painful swellings in the groin. These swellings are enlarged lymph nodes. Lymph nodes? What are they? Lymph nodes are part of the immune system which protects us from the ravages of invading germs whether they be bacteria or viruses. If we are successful in waging war against such germs, then we feel fine and have few signs of the battle. In other, more severe cases, our body has to call on each and every component of our defence system for aid. The lymph nodes produce specialized white blood cells called lymphocytes. After being "manufactured" in the lymph node, the lymphocytes move into the bloodstream so they can meet the foreign, invading germs. The lymphocytes are very efficient as they surround and gobble up the invaders. When our body has to produce billions of lymphocytes at short notice, the lymph nodes work overtime and thus become enlarged and tender. This explain the tender, swollen lymph nodes which are seen with herpes and many other infections. A non-STD example we are all familiar with are the small, tender lumps in our necks which accompany a sore throat. Again, these lymph nodes are testimony to our battle with the bacteria causing the throat infection.

The primary herpes attack lasts from one to three weeks. Is that the end of it? For some people the answer is yes, but as mentioned earlier, about two-thirds of the people who have had a primary attack will have a recurrence.

Can herpes cause other problems? Yes, it can. One complication concerns the newborn child. If the mother has herpes in the last few weeks of pregnancy, there is a chance that the baby will come into contact with the infection during its passage through the birth canal. The herpes virus tends to "hang out" around the cervix (the neck of the womb) and so, if the virus is present at the time of birth there is a good chance that the baby will become infected. The same applies if the lesions due to herpes are active in the area of the vagina. Fortunately, in the majority of cases where a woman has had the virus, it takes a quiet "snooze" and lies low, so there is relatively little chance of the baby becoming infected. Herpes in the newborn is associated with serious complications including infection of the brain, which may result in mental retardation or even the death of the child. In such situations, delivery by caesarian section can avert this problem. If a woman has a history of herpes, it is now possible for her physician to carry out tests for the virus during the last few months of the pregnancy. If these tests show the virus to be present then delivery by caesarian section would be indicated. Although herpes is a relatively common infection, complications in the newborn are rare. Some authorities have estimated the risk as one in every twenty thousand deliveries. So, a pregnant woman with a history of herpes really has little to worry about, although she should inform her obstetrician of her history early in the pregnancy. Also, the development of new drugs has had an impact as far as the treatment of herpes in the newborn is concerned. The problem should be kept in perspective. For example, between 1973 and 1980, only 66 cases of herpes in the newborn were reported in Great Britain.

Anything else? Yes. Herpes genitalis has been linked to cancer of the cervix. This does not mean to say that herpes causes this cancer. In fact, at the present time we do not know the "cause" of this type of cancer. Either way, it makes sense for any woman who has a history of herpes genitalis to have a regular "Pap" (cancer "smear") test. The same recommendation applies to women who do not have herpes genitalis but whose partners have a history of the infection.

HOW COMMON IS HERPES?

Jim, Jill, Jenny and Paul,
The thin, the fat, the short, the tall,
Tiny viruses like us all.

Herpes is very common. Although it is not easy to prove, there is a certain body of opinion which believes that herpes is increasing in incidence. By means of blood test surveys carried out in large communities, there is some evidence to show that a significant number of people have come into contact with the herpes virus at some time in their lives. Of course, as mentioned previously, many of these individuals may have received the infection through an innocent kiss from a person who had a cold sore on the lip, rather than through sexual intercourse. As might be expected, younger children show evidence of infection with herpes virus type I, while sexually active people show signs of coming into contact with the herpes type II virus. However, most individuals remain asymptomatic, that is, they become infected but develop no obvious signs or symptoms.

The infection was well known to the Romans, particularly in the form of cold sores on the lips. However, for many years it was thought that women were immune to the infection. We now know that both females and males are good candidates for herpes.

It is difficult to put an exact number to the cases that occur because herpes is not a notifiable infection. That is, unlike some other infectious diseases, like tuberculosis and gonorrhea, it is not usual to notify the health authorities of any cases that come to light. However, it has been estimated that in the U.S.A. over ten million people are infected with the herpes virus, though most are asymptomatic. Also, it is thought that every year up to half a million individuals have a first episode of herpes.

As far as most countries are concerned, it seems that herpes is present in epidemic proportions, particularly in the 15 to 30 year age group.

FOOD FOR THOUGHT

One-third of the number of people who have a first attack of herpes have no recurrences and have no more trouble with the infection. Lucky people, you might say, but it is not just a matter of luck. The key word is *immunity.* To be immune to an infection means that you are protected from getting that particular disease. We all remember those jabs in the arm which immunized us against a variety of childhood diseases. Such immunization enabled us to develop certain chemicals called *antibodies* which would attack the infections and so protect us against the diseases.

Such protection is only possible if our immune system fights the infection in question. If there is no response from the immune system, the infection takes over and gives us a miserable time. In the case of people who have no recurrences of herpes, their immune system has effectively battled the virus. In those individuals who are troubled with further episodes, it appears that the herpes virus can overcome the efforts of their immune systems. Further research is needed on this aspect. It is hoped that the findings of this research will enable us to eradicate herpes.

WHAT CAN CAUSE HERPES TO RECUR?

As you know by now, the herpes virus can lie low for months or even years, then suddenly flare up. What causes this? This aspect of research has been rather neglected, but we do have some idea of a few of the factors which may trigger a recurrence. Stress is known to be capable of precipitating an attack. Other factors include sexual intercourse, sunlight, fevers, and injury. Many other aspects of immunity play an important part, but further research is needed for these to be clarified. For example, it is well known that fit people find it easier to fight off infections. Diet is recognized as having an influence on our immune systems, and some authorities suspect that all the chemical "junk" we consume in the form of additives and preservatives may influence our defence reactions to various illnesses, including herpes.

HOW IS HERPES DIAGNOSED?

A history of recurrent blisters, sores or similar skin lesions in the genital area is suggestive of herpes genitalis. As is the case with all STD, it is essential that the person in question visit a physician or local STD clinic so that a full examination and the proper laboratory tests may be carried out. In all cases it is important to exclude other STD, particularly syphilis and gonorrhea. Remember, STD are sociable infections which like to travel about in two or threes. It is also wise for the patient's sexual partner to have a full check-up.

Although one might have a good idea that a particular skin lesion is herpes, one can only confirm the diagnosis using special tests. Unfortunately, these are not available in all laboratories. The virus can be grown in the lab using tissue cultures. These tests, however, take time to carry out and cannot be used to make a quick diagnosis. Blood tests are also available, but these may also be positive where there is a past history of herpes. The Pap test, used to detect cancer of the cervix, may also indicate the presence of herpes in women.

CAN HERPES BE TREATED?

Over the years people have tried virtually every remedy under the sun for the treatment of herpes. All of these treatments had one distinguishing feature in common: they didn't have any obvious effect on the infection.

In the early 1800s, Thomas Bateman, a progressive physician working in Yorkshire, England, was able to proffer the sound advice: "Avoid that which is moist and irritable." Sir Jonathon Hutchinson, born in 1828, a surgeon of international repute who saw over a million patients with syphilis, prescribed arsenic applications for herpes. Born in 1832, Professor Jean-Alfred Fournier, a leading teacher at the distinguished clinic at the Hôpital St. Louis in Paris, devoted most of his life to the study of syphilis. For herpes he recommended "starch, poultices, cold creams and regular applications of bismuth and talc." In more recent times, a wide assortment of remedies have been used, including local applications of ether, chloroform, and various antiseptics. The application of various dyes followed by "light" treatment has also been tried, but has now been discontinued because of adverse effects. Such treatments have little impact on the condition. Penicillin and other antibiotics also have no effect on the herpes virus.

Some antiviral agents such as idoxuridine have been incorporated into ointments and these preparations appear to shorten the course of the disease. Various vaccinations, including the smallpox vaccination, have also been used, but there is little evidence to show that such procedures have any impact on the infections, and they may be accompanied by serious side effects. It is hoped that a specific vaccine will be developed in the future.

"Government approves new drug to ease herpes pain." So reads the headline on the front page of the local paper. That sounds rather reassuring. Can we now forget the ravages of herpes? Not yet. A drug, said to be capable of easing the symptoms of herpes genitalis, has now been cleared for use in the U.S.A. and Canada. The key phrase here is "easing the symptoms": the drug cannot cure or prevent herpes. It is claimed that when used in the early stages of the disease, the outcome will be less painful. The drug is based on the chemical acyclovir, and is available as an ointment. The compound does not appear to influence the course or recurrences of the infection.

How about general measures? Frequent baths have a part to play. The sores or burst blisters of herpes should be kept dry and clean. Soaking the affected part in a weak salt solution has a soothing effect. (Two teaspoonsful of ordinary table salt are dissolved in a litre of water.) Cotton underwear, which allows the skin to "breathe" is preferable to synthetic materials.

Sexual intercourse should be avoided until all the lesions have completely healed. Any sexual partners should also have a check-up. What if you are involved in a relationship with someone who suffers from herpes? The same guideline applies — when the sores of herpes are present, sex should be avoided. Or, if the person in question feels an attack of herpes coming on, then it would be a very good idea to abstain from sex until the lesions have fully disappeared. Do contraceptives offer any protection? In general, the answer is no as far as herpes is concerned. The virus thrives in the presence of most contraceptives.

How about the condom? This type of contraception may offer very slight protection but remember, the herpes virus is so small that it can penetrate the structure of the condom with ease. So, we are back to square one – if sores are present, avoid sexual intercourse until the lesions have cleared.

What about the link between herpes and stress? Obviously such an aspect is very important in any relationship. It is hard to prove, but stress appears to play an important part in the recurrences of herpes. Unfortunately, many people with herpes become depressed and unduly miserable. A shame! The stress due to feeling this way may make the person susceptible to further episodes. Stress can take many forms. You may be worried about school work or "not getting along" with your friends or your family. You can be worried for a hundred other reasons. Being able to relax, keeping fit and in good shape are some measures which are useful in warding off stress. Both partners should feel comfortable when discussing herpes, or any other STD, for that matter. The person with herpes should not be treated as a social "outcast." Being optimistic helps. A *positive* approach to the infection has been shown in some studies to cut the number of recurrent episodes of herpes down by 50%.

Herpes may occasionally be transmitted to the eye. So, if the skin lesions are handled, it makes sense to wash one's hands well with soap and water.

Organizations offering help include:

In Canada:

REACH
(Research, Education & Assistance for Canadians with Herpes)
P.O.Box 70
Station G
Toronto, Ontario Canada M4M 3E8

In the United States:

HELP
P.O.Box 100
Palo Alto, California 94320

In the U.K.:

THE HERPES ASSOCIATION
c/o Spare Rib
27 Clerkenwell Close
London EC1, England

CHAPTER 8

A TRIO OF NASTIES: YEAST INFECTIONS, GENITAL WARTS AND TRICHOMONIASIS

Misery acquaints a man with strange bedfellows.
— Shakespeare

THE STORY OF YEAST INFECTIONS

Yeasts are plants which belong to the fungi family. Yeast produces alcohol and carbon dioxide from sugar and is used in brewing alcohol and in breadmaking. Yeast lacks the green pigment *chlorophyll* which is used by most plants to manufacture food with the aid of sunlight. So yeast and other fungi feed off others. Some fungi, such as toadstools and mushrooms, are quite obvious to the naked eye, but others such as yeasts, can only be observed with the assistance of a microscope. We consider some fungi as good and others as bad. Obviously, it is very useful to have yeast to make our bread rise or to use it in brewing wines. On the other hand, some fungi are capable of causing serious infections, particularly in people who have a weak immune system. You may be familiar with the fact that women often get yeast infections; men can also become infected, though in most instances they feel fine and have no symptoms. Fortunately, the yeast we are going to discuss in this chapter is usually more of a nuisance than a serious threat to health.

WHAT'S IN A NAME?

There are many different types of yeast. The one we are interested in is called *Candida albicans*. It is also known as "thrush," "yeast," or "monilia." For convenience, we will use the term yeast. This organism is commonly found in humans, and in most cases the yeast is not transmitted sexually. It is already there; it is only when environmental conditions in the vagina change that the yeast multiplies and upsets the balance. Yeast is a normal inhabitant of the mouths and bowels of millions of individuals. In the majority of cases it causes no trouble and has no symptoms.

YEAST PREFERS FEMALES

When yeast does decide to be a nuisance, it causes problems in females rather than males. Symptoms in males are relatively rare, although many males carry the infection without knowing it.

Why is it that many women may have yeast present in the vagina, yet the organism causes few problems? At this point it should be mentioned that our bodies are host to various bacteria and fungi which appear to co-exist peacefully with us. For many years very little was known about the microbes which inhabit the normal vagina. In 1892, Albert Doderlein studied the problem and discovered that the normal vagina contains groups of bacteria which maintain a level of lactic acid in the vagina. This acts as a partial defence against infection. Unfortunately, these bacteria do not offer complete protection against invading microbes. Anything which disturbs the delicate balance of optimum acidity in the vagina (such as pregnancy, antibiotics or uncontrolled diabetes), enables yeast and other microbes to grow undisturbed. More on this later. The group of bacteria which are "normal" or "welcome" inhabitants of the vagina are called *Doderlein's bacilli*.

WHAT CAN YEAST DO?

Yeast is fine in bread and wine
But socially speaking, yeast's a beast

Yeast is a common cause of vaginal discharge in females, but as previously mentioned, in many instances the organism is not present as an STD.

The vaginal discharge caused by yeast is usually white in colour and is said to resemble cottage cheese in appearance. The discharge is often associated with discomfort or irritation around the vagina. This irritation may be associated with pain on passing the urine. Sometimes there is pain on intercourse (which goes under the name of *dyspareunia*). Often the discharge comes and goes.

IS ANYONE ELSE INVOLVED?

If a pregnant woman has a vaginal yeast infection there is a chance that the newborn baby may become infected. Usually this takes the form of a mild mouth infection. This is a relatively common occurrence which causes no serious problems and responds well to specific anti-fungal treatment.

HOW IS YEAST DIAGNOSED?

The typical appearance of yeast is easily diagnosed when a small amount of the discharge is examined under the microscope. For a more accurate and scientific answer, the yeast can also be grown on a special "food" (called Sabouraud's medium) where large colonies of the yeast then become visible to the naked eye. This is akin to the blue and green patches which are seen on mouldy bread (these are also caused by fungi).

A REMINDER

Although yeast is a common inhabitant in most of our bodies, it should be remembered that on occasions the organism is transmitted sexually. So if a person thinks that she or he may have acquired a yeast in this way it makes sense to have a thorough check-up. This is to exclude other STD since yeast infections may co-exist with other members of the STD family. Any sexual partners should also be checked out.

WHAT MAKES YEAST GROW?

Anything which disturbs the level of acidity in the vagina tends to encourage the growth of yeast. For example, antibiotics, particularly the newer, more powerful types, tend to discourage the multiplication of the beneficial *Doderlein bacteria*. So it is not surprising to find that individuals who take antibiotics for extended periods of time are very susceptible to yeast infections.

Hormones (chemicals produced by living cells which have a specific effect on other living cells) also play a part. Synthetic hormones such as those used in the oral contraceptive (the pill) and cortisone may also promote the growth of yeast infections. The hormonal changes that happen in pregnancy act in a similar way.

It is well recognized that diabetics are susceptible to yeast infections since yeasts flourish where there is an excess of sugar in the body. Other conditions which result in a lowered resistance to infection tend to facilitate the growth of yeast as well. So, if a person suffers from recurrent yeast infections, this may be a sign of another underlying cause. It is always important to have a thorough examination to exclude such a cause.

TREATMENT

So many people have been heard to wail
"Expensive treatment has been to no avail"

In the majority of cases yeast infections are relatively easy to get rid of. However, they do have a tendency to recur. In all cases it is essential to detect any underlying cause and to exclude other causes of a vaginal discharge. The majority of such discharges are not due to STD, but it is always important to rule out an STD by the appropriate tests. Even with adequate therapy, some women appear to be unduly prone to yeast infections. In such cases, one possible explanation is that the male partner may be carrying the yeast organism on his penis without being aware of it and the woman keeps being re-infected.

Several anti-fungal preparations are available to treat this condition. Some are in cream form and some are in tablet form. Both forms of treatment are intended for use in the vagina. The cream can also be used to treat yeast infections of the penis. Sexual intercourse should be avoided until both partners have been treated. Synthetic underwear should be replaced by cotton underwear which allows the skin to "breathe."

GENITAL WARTS

"Say, what is dead cats good for, Huck?"
"Good for? Cure warts with"
— Mark Twain

Tom Sawyer and Huckleberry Finn's view of warts was a testimony to the lack of success humans have had in their battles against the common wart. The many recipes for the successful removal of warts to be found in the folklore of many countries only shows how ineffective conventional remedies were. Many believed the warts to be souvenirs marking a visit from a witch or evil spirit. In such cases divining rods and "words of magic" were used to cleanse the skin. Others used carrot "poultices." Ointments incorporating dried worms, foxes' lungs, or oil of ants were brought into the act. Concoctions containing "black tops of crabs paws", jalap, cock's comb, fur and feathers also had their supporters. Such preparations were not cheap and competition was fierce amongst the sellers of such "cures."

Warts have always had a place in history and even Oliver Cromwell (1599-1658) had strong views on the subject. When he was to have his portrait painted he instructed the painter, "Mr. Lely, I desire you would use all your skill to paint my picture truly like me, and not to flatter me at all: but remark all these roughnesses, pimples and warts . . ."

Such references are to the common warts which most of us have had on our hands from time to time. However, there is another type of wart which is spread sexually and so belongs to the STD family.

WHAT ARE WARTS?

Warts are small, firm protruberances on the skin. We have mentioned the common warts of the hand which are not usually transmitted sexually. Another type of wart that many of us are familiar with is the plantar wart, which is frequently found in

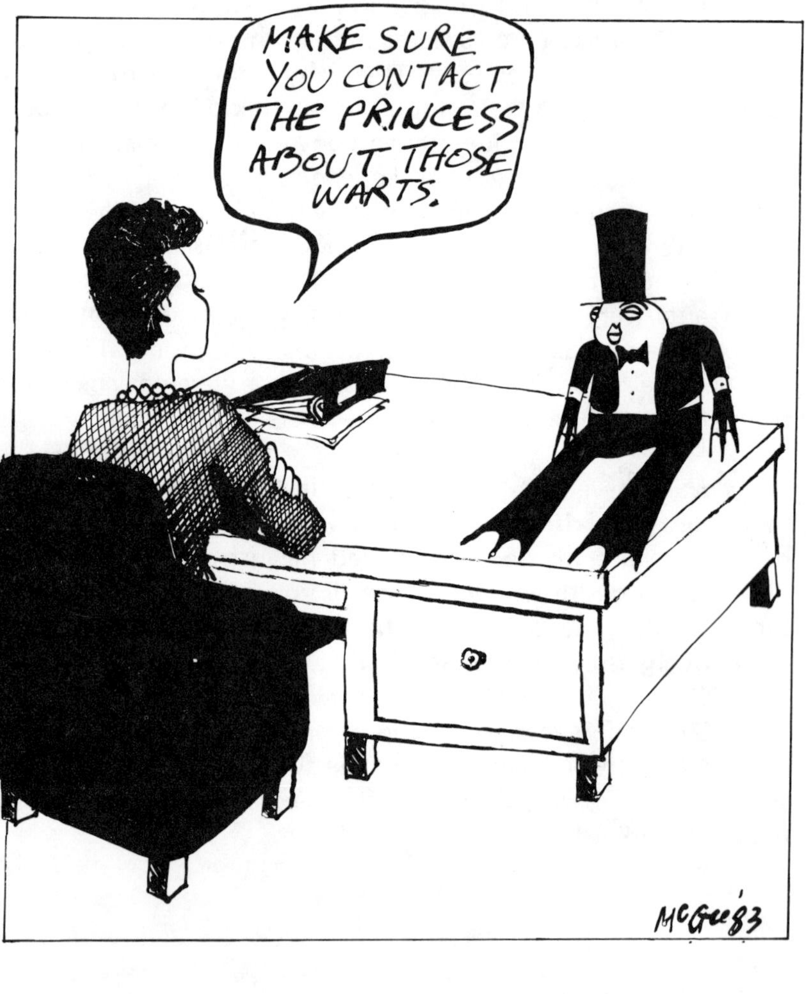
MAKE SURE YOU CONTACT THE PRINCESS ABOUT THOSE WARTS.
McGee '83

In general, the typical appearance of genital warts make them easy to diagnose.

the sole of the foot. This can make walking difficult, and has been associated with swimming pools and gyms. Again, this type of wart is not sexually transmitted.

WHAT CAUSES WARTS?

Warts are caused by the *papilloma* virus. This virus can only be seen with the aid of powerful electron microscopes. Warts are an infection and they can be easily spread.

WHERE DOES SEX COME IN?

Some wart-forming viruses have a preference for the genital area. These *genital warts* are sexually transmitted and affect both males and females. In males they usually settle for the penis and in females they prefer the skin around the vagina and the vagina, itself. Warts are sometimes found in the anal area, particularly in gay males. The warts may occur in twos and threes, but on other occasions they may be more numerous.

Do these STD cause many problems? On the whole, warts are more of a nuisance than a serious problem. However, on rare occasions, if a pregnant woman suffers from vaginal warts, there is a chance that the newborn baby will be affected. In such instances the baby's larynx (voicebox) may be involved.

DIAGNOSIS

In general, the typical appearance of genital warts make them easy to diagnose. In all cases it is important to exclude the presence of other STD. An association with other STD, especially gonorrhea and yeast infections, is not uncommon. Also, it is essential to check the sexual partner for warts and other STD. In some studies, it has been shown that 60% of the partners of individuals with genital warts had a history of the same condition.

Warts may mimic other skin diseases and if there is any doubt about the diagnosis, then a *biopsy* should be carried out. This involves examining a small piece of the wart under the microscope to confirm the diagnosis.

INCUBATION PERIOD

What is the incubation period for genital warts? On the average, it is about four to six months, although it can last as long as one year.

TREATING WARTS

Do they go away on their own? In some cases they do. Modern science has so far failed to come up with a safe, simple and effective method to cure genital warts. At the present time such techniques as *freezing* the warts with liquid nitrogen or *cauterizing* (burning them) have been tried, but the results are sometimes disappointing.

A plant extract called podophyllin is also used to treat the lesions. However, this has potentially serious adverse effects and should only be used under the direct supervision of a physician or clinic. The application is left on for several hours and then washed off. This procedure may need to be repeated once or twice a week for several weeks. It must not be used on pregnant women because of the potential risks involved.

All in all we are still awaiting the day when our leading virologists and research workers will come up with the cure for warts. The individual who finds a safe, cheap and effective way to eliminate them may well be thought worthy of a Nobel prize by the millions of people who get warts.

CAN TV CAUSE TROUBLE?

It certainly can! We're not talking about television here, we're dealing with another STD called trichomoniasis. This infection is caused by a small microorganism called *Trichomonas vaginalis* (TV). The chances are that most of you will not have heard of this condition. Even so, TV is very popular and infects millions of people, both females and males. Some authorities estimate that one out of every five sexually-active females will come into contact with the parasite at some time in her life. It is interesting to note that these same authorities provide no figures for males! However, by now the reader knows that "it takes two to tango" so we can safely assume that a large number of males also come into contact with TV.

TV = TRICHOMONAS VAGINALIS

The TV organism is pear-shaped and is easily observed under the microscope. Using several hair-like projections called flagella, it swims and wiggles around for hours on end. TV was first discovered by a researcher named Donné in the year 1836.

WHAT DOES TV DO?

Firstly, it should be said that TV often causes no problems. In other instances, like the other STD bedfellows referred to earlier in this chapter, TV can really be a nuisance. In females, it may cause an offensive, yellow vaginal discharge which is associated with great irritation and discomfort. Pain on sexual intercourse and on passing the urine are not uncommon. Most males who carry TV remain free from symptoms, sometimes though, there can be a discharge from the penis and discomfort on urinating.

INCUBATION PERIOD

Jim has TV but feels just fine. How long will it be before his new girlfriend Janice shows signs that Jim has passed this infection on to her? Remember, she may not necessarily pick up the infection at all. If Jim regularly uses a condom, the chance of the organism being passed on to her is significantly reduced. If Janice does acquire TV, it will show up from three days to three weeks later.

HOW DO I KNOW IF I HAVE IT?

A small drop of the discharge is examined under the microscope and the typical appearance of the wiggling, pear-shaped TV confirms the diagnosis. The organism can sometimes be detected on a Pap smear. It is usually impossible to detect the organism in males. Ordinarily, TV causes few or no symptoms in males. It appears to "hang out" in the secretory fluid of the prostate gland — samples of the fluid are hard to obtain in routine clinical practice. That's why the test for TV is usually negative in males. It is not a common cause of a urethral discharge in males. Needless to say, it is always important to exclude other STD, particularly gonorrhea. Any sexual partners should also have an STD check-up.

TREATING TV

Several drugs are available for the treatment of TV. One popular preparation is called *metronidazole*. It may be taken orally in a single dose. However, there are potential adverse effects and the drug must be given under medical supervision. Both the patient and her or his sexual partner should be treated at the same time, and both parties should abstain from intercourse until a cure has been confirmed by follow-up tests. Certain laboratory studies have raised some questions about the safety of metronidazole. Because of the potential side effects, the drug should not be used during pregnancy.

CHAPTER 9

LICE AND CREEPY CRAWLIES: SOME COMMON AND SOME EXOTIC SEXUALLY TRANSMITTED DISEASES

LOUSY LICE

If it is alive and small, chances are it can crawl.

A louse is a wingless insect with six legs. In Tudor times the aristocrats carried long-handled combs so that they could scratch their backs and so ease the irritation caused by lice. These people rarely bathed; they thought it was bad for their health. Today, people who are clean don't get lice, do they? Yes they do!

Many people find it hard to believe that lice are alive and kicking in this modern age. However, these hardy insects continue to infest millions of humans throughout the world.

Most people view the human louse with contempt and disdain. We still use the adjective "lousy" or call someone who acts badly a "louse." Lice respect no rank or person, and in days gone by they infested the royalty, the court nobility and the "commoners" alike. Lice have played starring roles in major plagues and pestilences throughout history and have thus been responsible for millions of deaths. The lice did this by giving a "piggy-back" ride to such serious infections as typhus (also known as gaol fever).

WHY ARE LICE A NUISANCE?

Although our main concern is with the STD implications of lice, we will mention some of the other types that affect humans:

1. Crab lice ("crabs"): The crab louse is technically known as *Phthirus pubis.* This louse resembles the sea crab. As far as we know, it does not transmit any serious diseases to humans. This is the STD louse.
2. Head lice ("nits"): These lice inhabit the hairs of the head and spread easily in such places as schools. It is not an STD louse.
3. Body lice: These lice tend to live in clothing. They drift back to the human body whenever they feel hungry. In the past, they were the main carriers of typhus. This disease is still found in parts of Latin America, Asia and Africa. It also, is not an STD louse.

Now back to the crab louse. This creature lives in the genital area and is now classed as an STD. In most cases it is spread from person to person by sexual intercourse.

How large are crab lice? Each one is about one millimetre long. Using their rear legs, they attach themselves to the hair shafts in the genital area. The female lays about fifty eggs at a time and she attaches these to the hairs with a type of insect glue. The attached eggs are called nits. It should be stressed again that the nits that appear on the *head* are *not* an STD.

The eggs of the crab louse hatch in seven to ten days. The average life span of the female louse is some thirty-five days; the male insect dies even sooner. Although there is no true incubation period, if a person comes into contact with someone carrying crab lice, it will probably be about two to four weeks before they notice anything.

WHAT DO CRABS DO?

Crab lice are a nuisance because they like to bite us and suck our blood. This is how they survive and it is these bites that cause itching and irritation. After a juicy meal they can be seen by the naked eye as small, red pinheads. The nits are also visible.

TAKE A LOOK

So, how does a person know whether they have crabs or not? By taking a look! Seeing is believing. All recent sexual partners should also be checked out for the condition, and all parties should make sure that no other STD are present by having the appropriate tests carried out.

GETTING RID OF CRABS

Merely washing them off is not sufficient. Many special preparations are available in the form of lotions for treating the condition. Some popular preparations contain a chemical called gamma benzene hexachloride. However, it is now known that such chemicals may be absorbed through the skin and may spread to the rest of the body. So many authorities recommend that this type of preparation not be used on young children or pregnant women. This is not really a problem since alternative treatment is available.

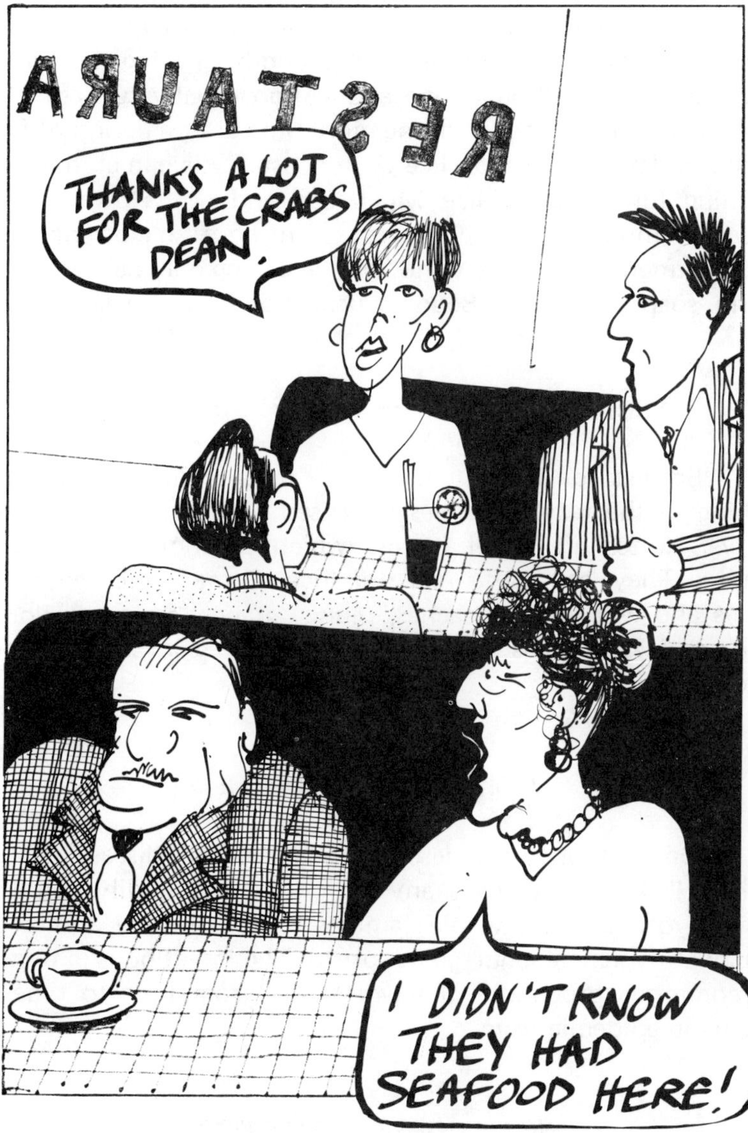
THANKS A LOT FOR THE CRABS DEAN.
I DIDN'T KNOW THEY HAD SEAFOOD HERE!

The crab louse lives in the genital area and is now classed as an STD.

The lotion is applied to the affected area and it is also important to apply it to the surrounding area. After about eight or ten hours the lotion is washed off, and the dead lice and nits may be removed with a fine-toothed comb. Shaving the hair is not necessary. Although one application usually suffices, the treatment may be repeated one more time after a period of five to seven days. These crab lice do not usually live in clothing or bedding (unlike body lice which can and do). However, for peace of mind, most people prefer to put on fresh clothing after the treatment. If necessary the "old" clothing may be washed in warm soap and water. Bedding need not be discarded either.

SCABIES, ANOTHER CREEPY-CRAWLY

Scabies, or the "itch," is the most common cause of itching in the world. Scabies is caused by the mite *Sarcoptes scabiei.* Mites are small insects which belong to the spider family. They can be a real nuisance. Some prefer gourmet meals and will attack peaches, plums, grapes, grain and flour. The scabies mite has four pairs of legs and it loves to burrow into our skins.

A MITE TOO SOCIABLE

One authority has described scabies as a "disease of bedfellows." This mite loves any form of close bodily contact. Scabies often affect whole families; over-crowding and poor personal hygiene encourage its spread. The infection is extremely common throughout the world and from time to time it occurs in epidemic form.

WHAT DOES SCABIES DO?

Because of its ability to produce prolonged, intense itching in humans, scabies is often referred to as the "itch." How does it cause this? The female mite burrows into the skin and deposits her eggs. They hatch four days later. These eggs are the cause of the annoying itch. The burrows are mainly seen on the hands, wrists, and genital area, but other areas may be involved. Often the itching is more intense after exercise or after taking a warm bath, and night-time is often the occasion when the itching is a real problem.

How does a person know if they have scabies? The telltale scratch marks around the burrows are excellent clues. The diagnosis is confirmed by finding the mite in a "scraping" of the skin when seen under the microscope. The mite is usually not visible to the naked eye. If there is a history of sexual intercourse, it is wise to test for other STD. This applies, as always, to any sexual partners as well.

TREATING SCABIES

Showers and soaps have little effect. Lotions similar to those used in the treatment of crabs are usually successful in eliminating scabies. The lotion is applied to the entire body from the neck down. Twelve hours later, the application is washed off and a change of clothing should be made. Only the one application is required. As mentioned in the section on crabs, some of the preparations are not suitable for use on pregnant women or young children because of the potential adverse effects of the drug if it is absorbed through the skin. Many authorities prefer to treat the whole family as well as any sexual contacts.

MOLLUSCUM CONTAGIOSUM

It is only in recent years that *molluscum contagiosum* has been classed as an STD. This is a relatively common skin condition which is caused by a virus.

Anyone who has studied biology knows that molluscs are animals with a soft body protected by a hard shell. Oysters and snails, for example, are molluscs. The skin lesions of molluscum contagiosum tend to be soft and the disease is contagious, hence the name.

INCUBATION PERIOD

Molluscum contagiosum is a viral disease and the incubation period ranges from several weeks to several months. For a long time it was thought that the condition was acquired in swimming pools and Turkish baths, but it is now thought that in many cases the virus is spread as an STD.

WHAT DOES IT DO?

The virus causes small crops of bumpy lesions in the genital area or on the thighs. The skin lesions have a pearly appearance. It is always wise to exclude other STD through the appropriate tests. Usually, molluscum contagiosum causes little trouble. Treatment consists of either "scraping" the lesions out or of applying various chemicals to the surface of each bump.

HOT CLIMATES AND STD?

Some STD are associated with the tropics and subtropics. They are also seen in cooler countries, but less frequently. We will mention them briefly here, but most people will probably never come across them. The three we are concerned with are *Lymphogranuloma venereum, Chancroid,* and *Granuloma inguinale.*

LGV = LYMPHOGRANULOMA VENEREUM

Another long latin name! The interesting thing about LGV is that it is caused by a member of the Chlamydia trachomatis family. LGV is found in South America, the Caribbean, Africa and parts of Asia. It also tends to appear in international seaports, and it is imported into some countries by travellers.

INCUBATION PERIOD

The incubation period ranges from one to five weeks. The first sign is usually a sore in the genital area. Subsequent to this there is an enlargement of the lymph nodes in the groin. In some cases, headache, fever and joint pains are also experienced.

DIAGNOSING LGV

Diagnosis is based upon the patient's history and on blood tests for Chlamydia. A skin test was originally used, but has now been discontinued. Other STD should be excluded from the diagnosis, and all sexual partners should also be tested. Antibiotics, the tetracyclines, are used to treat LGV, but they need to be given over a period of two to three weeks. As with other STD, it is important for all the concerned parties to refrain from sexual intercourse until the cure has been confirmed by the appropriate follow-up tests.

CHANCROID (SOFT SORE)

Like LGV, chancroid is not commonly observed in the STD clinics in the western world. However, there have been outbreaks from time to time in such countries as Canada and Greenland. The infection is still present in tropical countries, and with the advent of jet-age travel it appears occasionally in countries throughout the world. In the past, it was associated with the seaports.

Haemophilus ducreyi, the bacteria causing chancroid, were discovered by the researcher Auguste Ducrey in 1889.

INCUBATION PERIOD

The incubation period ranges from two to seven days. The infection is associated with sores in the genital area and enlarged lymph nodes in the groin.

By now you will be aware that several STD are associated with the same signs and symptoms. For example, syphilis, LGV, herpes and chancroid are all associated with sores in the genital area and enlarged lymph nodes. Can you tell the difference between these lesions just by looking at them? The answer is no. This is why such STD can only be accurately diagnosed if the appropriate tests are carried out.

TREATING CHANCROID

Treatment is with antibiotics, such as tetracycline. These are given over a period of several weeks. As for other STD, follow-up tests are also indicated.

GRANULOMA INGUINALE

Granuloma inguinale is relatively rare in most countries. It is found in parts of Africa, Asia, and some Pacific Islands. There is some doubt as to whether it is a true STD. It is caused by an organism called *Donovania granulomatis* and the incubation period is between a few weeks and a few months.

The infection is associated with ulcers or "granulomatous" skin lesions. Diagnosis is by biopsy (taking a small piece of the skin lesion and examining it under the microscope). It has to be distinguished from other STD. Appropriate antibiotics taken over an extended period of time are the treatment.

CHAPTER 10

THE GAY LIFE AND SEXUALLY TRANSMITTED DISEASES

This chapter will deal with the STD implications for homosexuals (those people whose sexual preference is with others of their own sex).

DO GAY PEOPLE NEED TO WORRY ABOUT STD?

Old ideas do linger on. For many years it was commonly believed that gay people did not get STD. This is false. Remember, STD may be acquired by *any* sexually active person. In the majority of instances the risk for homosexuals is the same as for heterosexuals (those whose sexual preference is with members of the opposite sex). Yet, in the case of one or two specific infections, the risk for homosexuals is relatively high.

For many years people believed that women did not get STD. Of course, we now know that this is not true and that STD in females can be a real threat. On the other hand, STD in gay females (lesbians) is not usually a big problem. In fact, STD in lesbians is usually confined to infections such as trichomoniasis or yeast. Most STD are transmitted by penetration of the penis (into the vagina, for example). Since the sexual contact between lesbians is different, the risk of spreading STD appears to be greatly reduced. Of course, bisexuals are exposed to, and are susceptible to all STD.

GAY MALES AND SYPHILIS

Although syphilis is not one of the most common of the STD, it is still one of the most serious. What with jet-age travel the infection manages to cross from country to country and from continent to continent. The World Health Organization has estimated that there are some fifty million cases of syphilis in the world each year. Many countries report one interesting, though unexplained, fact, namely: the majority of cases of syphilis occur in gay males. It is dangerous to make generalizations about STD and at this time no one is sure why gay males seem to be so highly susceptible to syphilis.

In many international cities, such as Rome, New York, Amsterdam and London, the proportion of gay males with this infection is unduly high. In 1980 in the U.S.A. some twenty-seven thousand cases of syphilis were notified to the health authorities. Of this number, just over twenty thousand cases involved males. How many of these men were gay is unknown, as the notification of infectious diseases does not demand that sexual preference be stated.

Most authorities now recommend that gay males have a check-up for this infection and other STD every three or four months. This policy enables the infection to be detected and treated in the early stages, thus preventing complications. In many countries the level of syphilis has remained constant and there is no reason why we should not be able to control this disease.

GAY MALES AND GONORRHEA

Remember how gonorrhea remained silent in the majority of females? Well, in gay males the infection also often prefers to lie low, particularly where the rectum and throat are concerned. Of course, the common symptoms of gonorrhea, such as discomfort on passing the urine and a discharge from the tip of the penis may also be present. Sometimes these two symptoms of discomfort and a discharge may be present in the rectum. Once again, a regular check-up for STD is a wise policy.

KILLER DISEASES?

Moriz Kaposi was a distinguished Hungarian skin specialist, born in 1837. He described the strange and rather rare skin tumour which is now known as Kaposi's Sarcoma. In most western countries this skin growth is very uncommon, but strangely enough, it is relatively common among people living in the African tropics, particularly near the equator. What's the connection between Kaposi's tumour and STD? In 1981, the first reports came out linking Kaposi's Sarcoma to young, gay males. This skin condition forms part of the AIDS syndrome which first appeared in New York and San Francisco; cities with large gay populations.

AIDS

AIDS = ACQUIRED IMMUNODEFICIENCY SYNDROME

This condition is also known as the GRID Syndrome; Gay Related Immunodeficiency. Remember the defence or immune system which protects us from invading microbes? In the case of AIDS, the defence system fails to function and the body is thus left open to all kinds of infection. If the immune system cannot do its job, what happens? For starters, relatively minor infections, such as sore throats, can get out of hand and drag on and on. In the case of a chest infection such as pneumonia, the results may be fatal. The condition, associated with Kaposi's Sarcoma, is also linked with a rare form of pneumonia caused by a parasite named *Pneumocystis carinii.* There have been reports of AIDS in women, children and in non-gay males. The onset of this disease is not very noticeable, there is increasing fatigue, a gradual loss of weight, fever and a general feeling of being unwell.

What causes this baffling disease? Nobody really knows, but a virus called *Cytomegalovirus* and various street drugs, such as amylnitrate, have been incriminated. AIDS has been associated with people who abuse amylnitrate — this does not mean to say that the drug causes AIDS. Such viruses and drugs may impair the body's response to infection. Or, in other words, the immune or defence system is weakened so that infections can rapidly gain a hold.

IS AIDS COMMON?

Fortunately, it is not that common. Up to now, just over five hundred cases have been reported in the U.S.A. Some of these have been associated with fatalities. Other countries have reported a handful of cases. On the other hand, many cases may well have been overlooked or dismissed. Various drugs have been used to treat the condition but they have not always been successful.

LOVERS AND LIVERS

That young man has a secret way,
pecooliar to himself,
of getting at his heart, and at his liver.
— Charles Dickens

Most people are aware that alcohol can damage the liver. Can other conditions do the same thing?

We all have a large precious organ called the liver. In adults it tips the scales at about six kilograms (about thirteen pounds). What does it do? Working twenty-four hours a day, it manufactures various chemicals, such as bile salts which are needed for digestion. It stores some vitamins, such as B_{12} and it helps to regulate the sugar levels in our blood. The liver also destroys various poisons which are produced by or introduced into our bodies. In short, it functions as a chemical factory which is indispensable to life. Any chemicals or microbes which cause this factory to shut down will harm our health. So what's the connection between lovers and livers? Read on.

HEPATITIS

Hepar — the Greek word for liver. *Itis* — inflammation. So, *hepatitis* means an inflammation of the liver. In the past if a person felt unwell, they were often said to feel "liverish".

Viruses are a common cause of hepatitis. Often the individual in question gets "jaundiced", that is, their skin takes on a sallow, yellow appearance. This is probably where the expression "feeling off-colour" came from. Two viruses called *Virus A* and *Virus B* are known to cause hepatitis, and each of these viruses *may* be transmitted by sexual means. Here, we are referring to hepatitis as an STD. Most cases of hepatitis are not due to STD. However, hepatitis in gay males tends to be linked with STD.

Hepatitis is associated with nausea, fatigue, fever, loss of appetite and sometimes jaundice. Recovery is slow, taking weeks or months, but most people do make a 100% recovery. However, about five out of every hundred people with hepatitis B may go on to develop long-term complications. Also, about ten out of every hundred people with type B hepatitis continue to carry the virus in their bodies.

It is now known that gay males have *up to ten times* the chance of acquiring type B hepatitis compared to other sexually active individuals.

Encouraging news is that a new vaccine appears to be effective in immunization against type B hepatitis. However, it is relatively expensive and it is not possible to immunize everyone at risk at the present time. It has been estimated that worldwide there are some two hundred million carriers of the hepatitis B virus. Many of these people are in the developing countries.

PARASITES

A *parasite* is a hanger-on; an animal or plant which lives on another and draws nourishment from it. We all carry various parasites in our bodies. For example, our mouths usually contain thousands of various bacteria and microorganisms which usually cause little or no trouble. Fungi live on our skin and various microbes inhabit our bodies.

Some people pick up the more exotic parasites when they visit the tropics. *Malaria* is a parasite which is transmitted to humans via the bite of an infected mosquito. Other parasites are present in contaminated food or water. Many people who go on exciting visits to tropical and sub-tropical countries soon develop "traveller's diarrhea" after a few days. In many cases such intestinal upsets are due to parasites. All in all, millions of people throughout the world harbour parasites in one form or another.

STD AND INTESTINAL PARASITES

It is now known that some of the intestinal parasites may be transmitted from person to person as an STD. Some U.S. studies have shown that in certain cities, 30% of the gay males may have acquired a parasite in this way. The parasites include *Entamoeba histolytica, giardia lamblia* and bacteria of the *Shigella* family. In such cases there are often no symptoms. Other times there may be diarrhea, abdominal cramps, lots of gas, or vague intestinal problems. It should be mentioned that most of these parasites can easily be detected and treatment is usually quite straightforward. As is the case with other STD, it is important that any partners be checked out and treated as necessary.

What is the best way to cover the above aspects of STD in gay males? There can be little doubt that a regular check-up for STD will go a long way towards controlling their main STD problems.

CHAPTER 11

REDUCING THE RISKS OF GETTING SEXUALLY TRANSMITTED DISEASES

REDUCING THE RISKS OF GETTING STD

If you can't be good, be careful.

Prevention is always preferable to a cure. It would be great to think that we could prevent STD. Unfortunately, at the present time we do not possess any magical vaccines against this family of communicable diseases. We can immunize against measles, mumps, polio, tetanus and diphtheria, but there is no vaccine for gonorrhea, syphilis, genital warts, or herpes. So, for the moment, no country has been able to eliminate STD from its population.

STD = STAY TENDERLY DEVOTED

However, there are a few ways to minimize the risk. Here's one idea: besides standing for *Sexually Transmitted Diseases*, the letters STD can also mean *Stay Tenderly Devoted*. Or, to put it another way, staying faithful to one's partner is a good way to avoid exposure to STD. Remember, it "takes two to tango!" You don't need a computer to figure out that the greater the number of partners you become sexually involved with (partners who may also have been involved with other partners and so on), the greater the risk of getting an STD.

DOES KEEPING CLEAN HELP?

How about simple personal hygiene? Keeping yourself clean is a good habit, but merely keeping clean and showering every day does not really offer any protection against STD. Remember, *anyone*, even nice, clean people, can get STD. It was once believed that washing down the genital area with soap and water after intercourse would reduce the chances of picking up any STD. In practice, this procedure probably does more for peace of mind than anything else. Some people have thought that urinating after intercourse can lessen the risk of infection. Again, such a procedure has no significant impact on the course of STD.

HOW ABOUT ANTISEPTICS?

Antiseptics should *not* be used to treat any real or imagined STD. Such chemicals can cause severe injury to the genitalia.

CONTRACEPTIVES AND STD

Do contraceptives have any effect? The condom (prophylactic, protective sheath, safe, rubber or French letter) does offer some protection against STD (particularly gonorrhea) in that it minimizes contact. The diaphragm and various contraceptive creams offer very slight protection by creating a "hostile environment" which may make it difficult for the STD organisms to survive. One important point to remember is that the oral contraceptive (the pill) and the intrauterine device (the IUD) do not offer any protection against STD.

ANTIBIOTICS AND STD

How about antibiotics and other medicines? By now you will have realized that antibiotics are not the answer to each and every illness which afflicts people. There is no one perfect medicine which can prevent STD. Taking a few antibiotic tablets every now and then in the hope that they will ward off STD is foolish. Not only will such medication interfere with tests for gonorrhea and syphilis, but it encourages the emergence of drug-resistant infections. Then, when you really need them, the antibiotics will be of little use.

HOW CAN YOU TELL IF SOMEONE HAS AN STD?

Can you tell if a person has an STD by looking at them? Of course not. All kinds of people may get STD. Also, many infections lie dormant, and so the person may be asymptomatic (feel fine). So, regarding that "casual" encounter, there is little way of knowing what is in store for you. Of course if the "partner-to-be" mentions that she or he has any kind of discharge, sore or any other sign of possible STD, advise them to have a check-up and don't have intercourse with them until they have done so and received an all clear sign. It is always worthwhile to keep in touch with recent sexual partners. Then, if they or you are diagnosed as having STD, it will be relatively easy for you to contact each other.

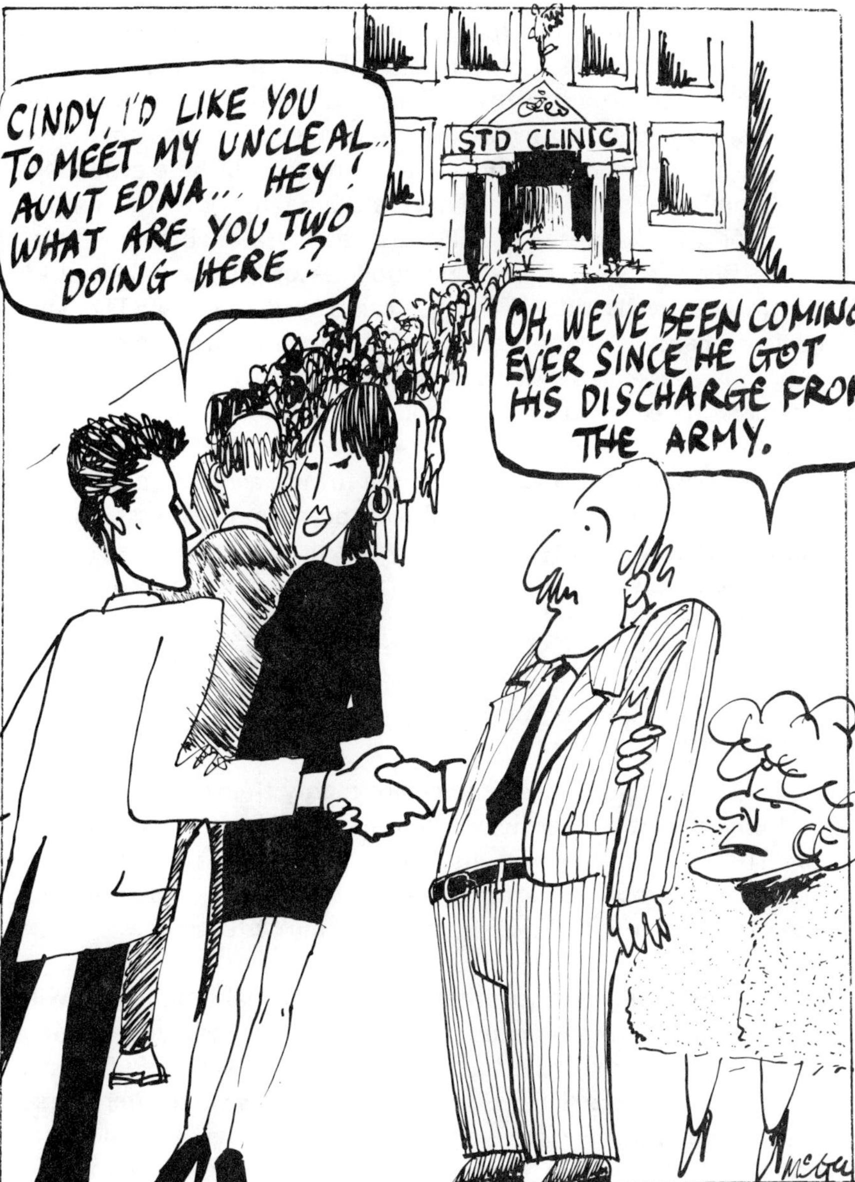
CINDY, I'D LIKE YOU TO MEET MY UNCLE AL... AUNT EDNA... HEY! WHAT ARE YOU TWO DOING HERE?
STD CLINIC
OH, WE'VE BEEN COMING EVER SINCE HE GOT HIS DISCHARGE FROM THE ARMY.

Even nice people get STD.

IF IN DOUBT, CHECK IT OUT

If a person thinks that she or he has, or may have, STD it makes sense to have a check-up. Unfortunately, many people are too shy or afraid to discuss the topic. These infections will not just go away by themselves, they must be dealt with. Some people will only go to a clinic if they're dragged there or if their symptoms are really severe. This is a shame, for now that simple tests for the diagnoses of STD are readily available and treatment is easy to take, there is no good reason why people should continue to walk around being "scared to death" of STD. The goal of health education about STD is to eradicate the mystery and stigma associated with these infections so that people can discuss and deal with them without embarassment.

It would be hoped that in the future, a visit to a clinic or physician to talk about an STD will be no more stressful than asking about a persistent cough. Many hospitals now have STD clinics and this has encouraged their acceptance by both professionals and the public.

WHAT HAPPENS IN AN STD CLINIC?

The staffs of these clinics are highly trained in their field and will go out of their way to ensure confidentiality and privacy. That means they will not phone your parents, your teachers or your boss and inform them of your visit. Remember, they are used to dealing with "embarassing" situations.

They will need to obtain a few personal details and will want to know why you are there. They will ask you routine questions. Do you have any symptoms of STD? (Perhaps a discharge or a sore?) Have you recently had sexual intercourse with a new partner? Do you use contraceptives? The nurse is not trying to pry into your private affairs, but is merely trying to obtain some basic information which will help the staff at the clinic to determine whether you have STD or not. Remember, many people who do consult with the staff of an STD clinic do not, in fact, have STD. Past studies have shown that in many countries up to half of the number of people who attend an STD clinic do not have STD.

In other words, many people go for advice, to be checked out, or to discuss a problem which has been keeping them awake at night.

After they have obtained some basic information from you, the physician or nurse will give you a physical examination to determine if any signs of STD are present. This examination will obviously focus on the genital area, but remember that STD may involve other parts of the body.

Then comes the question of tests. Some are uncomfortable, but isn't it preferable to undergo a small amount of discomfort than to walk around with gonorrhea? In males, a small cotton-swab is used to obtain a specimen from the tip of the penis. A smear from the orifice at the tip of the penis will be examined under the microscope to see if any evidence of gonorrhea, for example, is present. A sample of any discharge will be cultured to see if any STD germs grow.

In females, the examination is essentially a gynecological examination and a cotton swab is used to obtain a specimen from the cervix. Where indicated, specimens are also taken from the throats and rectums of both males and females.

The clinic staff will also recommend that blood tests, to exclude syphilis, be taken, and that a routine urine test be done.

Depending upon the test results, appropriate treatment will be prescribed. In many cases this will involve oral medicine (tablets to be taken by mouth). The use of injections is now less common and the majority of clinics prefer (as do their clients!) to use tablets in the treatment of gonorrhea. However, it is important to take the medication as directed and not to make up your own rules as you go along. Where an STD has been diagnosed and treated, the clinic will recommend that you return for a follow-up visit to confirm the cure. It is important to do this as some infections may be resistant to the treatment used and further medication, or even a change of medication, may be indicated. In the case of gonorrhea, most clinics will ask that you return some three to seven days later, after you have finished your medication.

"Hey! That's none of your business!" may be your first reaction when someone at the clinic asks you for details about your sexual partner. You're wrong, it is part of the clinic's business. Remember contact-tracing? If the clinic only treats you, it has only completed half the job. Your partner may still be walking around feeling fine, all the while harbouring gonorrhea. It is *important* that the clinic check your sexual partner. If gonorrhea were diagnosed, wouldn't you like to be told about it so you could also be treated?

On the other hand, some people with STD, even when they know that they have an infection, neglect to seek treatment, often due to guilt, anger or fear. Such an approach is to be strongly condemned. In addition to the implications of such behaviour for the community at large, such individuals also have a good chance of developing significant complications due to untreated STD. Telling partners when we develop STD is the only way we will have a chance of controlling STD in our communities.

ANXIETY, WORRY AND GUILT

What's the use of worrying?
It never was worthwhile,
So pack up your troubles in your old kit bag,
And smile, smile, smile.
— George Asaf (1880-1951)

By now you will have realized that many people, because of taboo, stigma and ignorance, worry needlessly about STD. In many cases just talking about the problem is sufficient to ease their anxiety. In other cases, a full range of STD tests may be required. Some people continue to worry unduly, even when their tests are negative and they've been informed that they are perfectly healthy. When feelings of guilt and anxiety run very deeply, psychiatric assistance may be indicated. This *venerophobia* is a product of our society's attitude to this group of diseases.

How often should a person have a check-up for STD? There is obviously no one correct answer to such a question. Each case must be judged individually. To review, if a person develops a discharge or a sore in the genital area, then obviously it's time for a check-up. Remember that STD are often acquired by people who frequently change sexual partners. So, the more partners, the greater the need for regular check-ups! Sexually active gay males appear to be at increased risk as far as several STD are concerned (syphilis and gonorrhea, for example), and so many authorities now recommend that such men have a check-up every three to six months. If a person is "going steady" with one regular partner and has no sexual contacts outside of this relationship, check-ups may be far less frequent.

Again, we have to keep the entire subject of STD in proper perspective. Nobody is recommending that every sexually active person should go around thinking of STD twenty-four hours a day! Life would be miserable if we did. Rather, we should be aware that these infections are a fact of everyday life, and that by using common sense, most people don't need to have undue fears about the subject.

PREVENTION OF STD

1. Remember, STD also stands for Stay Tenderly Devoted.
2. If you develop a discharge or a sore in the genital area, have a check-up with your physician or local STD clinic.

3. If you are anxious or worried about STD, do not hesitate to discuss the problem with others.
4. The use of condoms helps to reduce the risk of STD (not to mention unwanted pregnancy).
5. Do not share any STD treatment that has been prescribed for you. If your friends suspect they have an STD, advise them to go to an STD clinic.
6. If you are allergic to penicillin, you need have no worries regarding the treatment of STD. Good alternative antibiotics are readily available.
7. People who tend to have a number of sexual partners should have regular STD check-ups.

We seek him here, we seek him there,
We seek him everywhere.
Is he in heaven? Is he in hell?
That damned, elusive Pimpernel!
— Baroness Orczy (1865-1947)

The question of contact-tracing is an important one and should not be overlooked or forgotten. Unlike the Duchess in *Alice in Wonderland*, who thought that "If everybody minded their own business the world would go round a deal faster than it does" we now know that we have to bother with other people's affairs if STD is to be controlled and eradicated. Like the elusive Pimpernel, we seek the STD contact high and low.

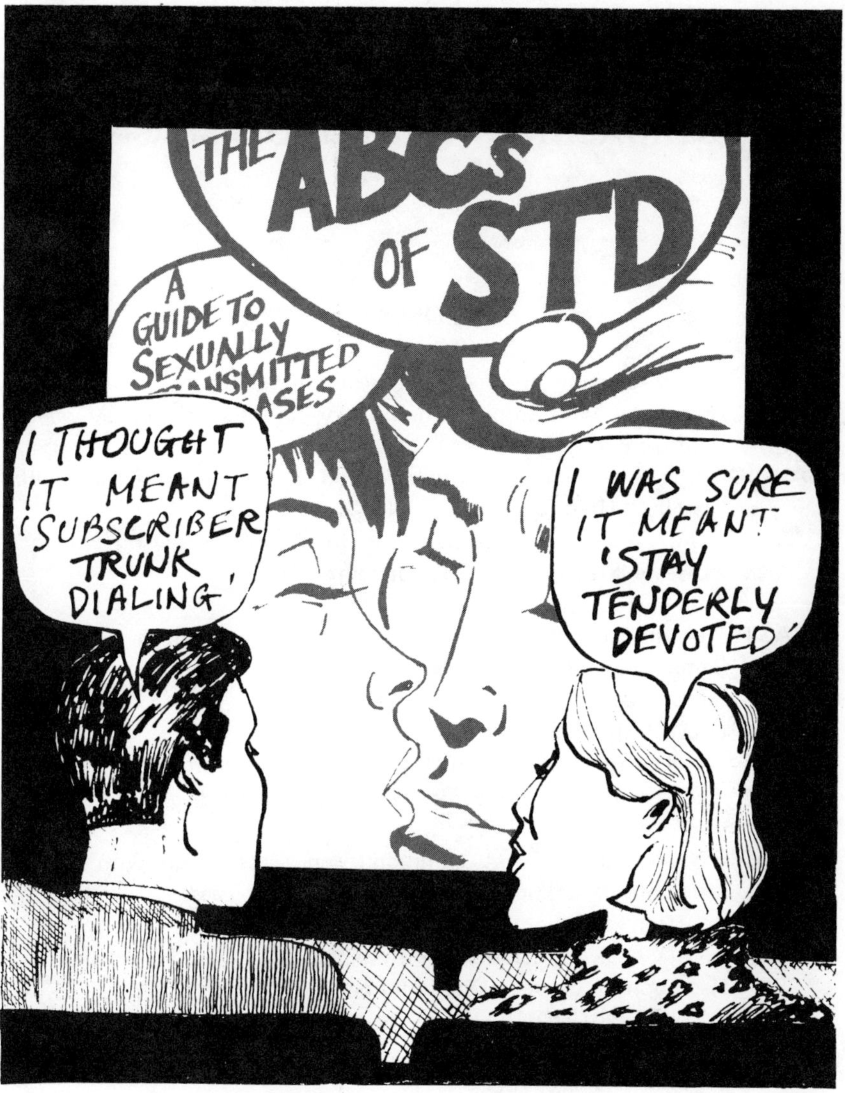
THE ABCs OF STD
A GUIDE TO SEXUALLY
I THOUGHT IT MEANT 'SUBSCRIBER TRUNK DIALING'
I WAS SURE IT MEANT 'STAY TENDERLY DEVOTED'

Staying faithful to one's partner is a good way to avoid STD.

THE ABCs OF STD
A NICE PERSON'S GLOSSARY OF SEXUALLY TRANSMITTED DISEASES

GLOSSARY

AIDS — Abbreviation for "Acquired Immuno-deficiency Syndrome." Associated with impaired immunity to infection in gay males. Relatively rare.

AMPICILLIN — A common antibiotic and a member of the penicillin "family." Used to treat several STD.

ASYMPTOMATIC — An adjective used to describe a person who has a disease but who has no obvious symptoms.

BACTERIA (Singular Bacterium) — Microscopic unicellular organisms. Some cause such diseases as gonorrhea and syphilis.

BALANITIS — An inflammation of the "tip" of the penis. Often associated with the fungus Candida albicans.

BIOPSY — The removal of a small piece of tissue from the body. This is then examined with a microscope to make a "diagnosis."

CANDIDA ALBICANS — A common fungus associated with vaginal infections. Also known as Thrush, Monilia or Yeast.

CERVIX — The "neck" or lower part of the uterus.

CHANCROID — A sexually-transmitted disease caused by a bacterium Haemophilus ducreyi. Mainly found in the tropics.

CHLAMYDIA TRACHOMATIS — A microscopic organism, which is associated with non-gonococcal urethritis (NGU) and lymphogranuloma venereum (LGV).

CRABS — Popular name for pubic lice.

DISCHARGE — A "flow of fluid." Used to describe an emission of fluid from the urethra or vagina.

DODERLEIN'S BACILLI – A group of bacteria which maintain the normal "acidity" of the vagina.

DONOVANIA GRANULOMATIS – The cause of Granuloma inguinale.

ECTOPIC PREGNANCY – A condition where the fertilized "egg" develops in an abnormal site outside the uterus.

EPIDEMIOLOGY – A science dealing with the distribution, incidence and control of disease in a given population.

FALLOPIAN TUBES – The "tubes" joining the ovaries to the uterus. A blockage of these may lead to difficulties in conceiving.

FTA-TEST – A specific blood test used to diagnose syphilis.

FUNGI – Lower plants which lack chlorophyll. Candida albicans is a fungus which is associated with vaginal infections.

GIARDIA LAMBLIA – A common intestinal parasite. Sometimes it may be sexually transmitted.

GONORRHEA – A common sexually transmitted disease. Also known as the "clap."

GRANULOMA INGUINALE – A sexually transmitted disease. Found mainly in the tropics.

GRIDS – Abbreviation for "Gay-related Immuno-deficiency Syndrome. Associated with impaired immunity in gay males. Now replaced by the term "AIDS."

GRANULOMA INGUINALE – A sexually transmitted disease. Found mainly in the tropics.

GRIDS – Abbreviation for "Gay-related Immuno-deficiency Syndrome. Associated with impaired immunity in gay males.

HAEMOPHILUS DUCREYI – The bacterium causing chancroid.

HEPATITIS – An inflammation of the liver. There are many causes including various chemicals and viruses.

HERPES GENITALIS – A common viral infection involving the genital region.

INCUBATION PERIOD – The time between first becoming "infected" and then developing signs of the disease.

INFLAMMATION – The response of the body to infection or chemical injury.

INTRAUTERINE DEVICE (IUD) – A contraceptive which "sits" inside the uterus.

JARISCH-HERXHEIMER REACTION — A "flu-like" reaction which sometimes occurs when syphilis is treated.

JAUNDICE — A yellow pigmentation of the skin which is associated with liver failure.

KAHN TEST — A blood test for syphilis. Now replaced by the VDRL test.

LICE — Small wingless insects. "Crab" lice are associated with the genital area.

LYMPHADENOPATHY — Enlargement of the lymph nodes. Occurs in association with various infectious diseases.

MOLLUSCUM CONTAGIOSUM — A skin condition which may be sexually transmitted. Caused by a pox virus.

MONILIA — A fungus associated with vaginal infections. Also known as Thrush, Candida albicans or Yeast.

NITS — Name used to describe the eggs laid by lice on human hair.

NON-GONOCOCCAL URETHRITIS (NGU) — An inflammation of the urethra. Often associated with Chlamydia trachomatis.

OPHTHALMIA NEONATORUM —An inflammation of the eyes of the newborn child. Associated with gonorrhea, Chlamydia trachomatis and other infections.

OVARIES — Paired female reproductive organs which produce "eggs."

PAP. TEST — The Papanicolaou smear or "Pap." test is used to detect early malignancy of the cervix.

PARASITE — An animal or plant which lives on another and obtains its nourishment from it.

PELVIC INFLAMMATORY DISEASE (PID) — An important complication of STD in females. Refers to an inflammation of the Fallopian tubes and pelvic organs.

PENICILLIN — A common antibiotic. Used to treat gonorrhea and syphilis.

PROSTATITIS — An inflammation of the prostate gland.

REITER'S DISEASE — A rare complication of non-gonococcal urethritis. Associated with inflammation of the joints and eyes. May also involve the skin.

SCABIES – A skin infestation caused by the mite Sarcoptes scabiei which produces intense irritation of the skin.

STD – Abbreviation for Sexually Transmitted Diseases.

SYPHILIS – A sexually transmitted disease caused by Treponema pallidum.

TETRACYCLINES – A group of common antibiotics. Some are used to treat STD.

THRUSH – A common fungus associated with vaginal discharge. Also called Candida albicans, Monilia or Yeast.

TRICHOMONAS VAGINALIS (TV) – A common unicellular organism associated with vaginal infections.

URETHRA – The channel along which urine passes from the bladder to the exterior.

URETHRITIS – An inflammation of the urethra.

VAGINITIS – Inflammation of the vagina.

VD – Short for Venereal Diseases. Now replaced by the term STD.

VDRL – Common blood test used to diagnose syphilis. Stands for "Venereal Disease Reference Laboratory."

VIRUSES – A group of sub-microscopic organisms that grow in living cells. Herpes genitalis and genital warts are caused by viruses.

WASSERMAN REACTION (WR) – The original test for syphilis. Now replaced by improved tests.

INDEX

Acyclovir, 73
Aids, 99
Antibodies, 70
Antibiotics, 15
Asymptomatic infections, 19

Bacteria, 15
Blood tests, 39

Candida albicans, 77
Chancre, 38
Chancroid, 95
Chlamydia Trachomatis, 45,
Clinics, 108
Contact tracing, 21
Contraceptives, 19
Crabs, 90

Dark field microscopy, 39
Doderlein's bacilli, 78
Drug resistant infections, 16
Dyspareunia, 78

Ectopic pregnancy, 56.
Epidemiology, 24
Eye infection, 27

Fallopian tubes, 27, 55

General paralysis of the insane (GPI), 35
Gonorrhea, 22
Gram stain, 23
Granuloma inguinale, 96

Haemophilus ducreyi, 95
Hepatitis, 101,
Herpes genitalis, 64

Idoxuridine, 73
Immunity, 70
Incubation period, 24
Infertility, 59

Jaundice, 101

Kissing, 7

Lice, 88
Lymph nodes, 67
Lymphocytes, 68
Lymphogranuloma venereum, 94

Metronidazole, 86
Molluscum contagiosum, 93
Monilia, 77

Neisseria gonorrhoeae, 23
Nits, 90
Non-gonococcal urethritis (NGU), 44
Ophthalmia, 27

Ovary, 55

Pap test, 28
Pelvic inflammatory disease (PID), 54
Penicillin, 42
Podophyllin, 84
PPNG, 31
Prostatitis, 26

Reiter's disease, 49

Salvarsan, 40
Scabies, 92
Statistics, 10
Stricture, 26
Syphilis, 32

Tetracycline, 52
Thrush, 77
Treponema pallidum, 36
Trichomonas vaginalis, 85

Urethritis, 44

VDRL test, 39
Venereal diseases, 3
Venereophobia, 111

Warts, 81
Wasserman test (WR), 39

Yeast infections, 77